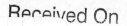

ALISO

Dance Me to the End

TEN MONTHS AND TEN DAYS WITH ALS

BRINDLE
AND GLASS

Edited by Kate Kennedy
Cover design by Tree Abraham
Interior design by Setareh Ashrafologhalai

LIBRARY AND ARCHIVES CANADA CATALOGUING IN PUBLICATION
Title: Dance me to the end : ten months and ten days with ALS / Alison
    Acheson.
Names: Acheson, Alison, 1964- author.
Identifiers: Canadiana 20190132728 | ISBN 9781927366868 (softcover)
Subjects: LCSH: Acheson, Alison, 1964- | LCSH: Acheson, Alison, 1964-—
    Family. | LCSH: Hatlelid, Marty, -2016—Health. | LCSH: Amyotrophic
    lateral sclerosis—Patients—Biography. | LCSH: Amyotrophic lateral
    sclerosis—Patients—Family relationships. | LCSH: Women caregivers—
    Biography. | LCGFT: Autobiographies.
Classification: LCC RC406.A24 A34 2019 | DDC 362.1968/390092—dc23

TouchWood Editions gratefully acknowledges that land on which we live and work is within the traditional territories of the Lkwungen (Esquimalt and Songhees), Malahat, Pacheedaht, Scia'new, T'Sou-ke and W̱SÁNEĆ (Pauquachin, Tsartlip, Tsawout, Tseycum) peoples.

We acknowledge the financial support of the Government of Canada through the Canada Book Fund and the Canada Council for the Arts, and of the Province of British Columbia through the British Columbia Arts Council and the Book Publishing Tax Credit.

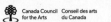 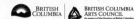

PRINTED IN CANADA AT FRIESENS

23 22 21 20 19   1 2 3 4 5

For our boys, now men

Two Years Earlier

It's a warm late afternoon in August
with an old friend getting married a second time, a
good time
I follow my husband as we trail across the grass

The wind off the river
relieves us from sun for a moment
A sense of homeostasis. I feel
happy

I recall one of our boys' favourite picture books, *Pizza for Breakfast*, and its closing line about being happy: "and this time they knew it"

Know happy, recognize it, memorize the feeling, sink it
into our bones
articulate, "This is happy"
and let the feeling imprint, allow ourselves
to move
toward it

2.

Goalposts

EARLY SUNDAY EVENING, last day of May, our family doctor called on the landline. On some level, I registered that must mean he wanted to talk with me specifically. He did. He asked if Marty and I could both come to his office at noon the next day. "This sounds serious," I said, and felt strangely, suddenly, disembodied. He didn't offer reassurance. Or reason. Just said he'd like to see us both. Together. The Team.

We ate dinner shortly after the phone call, my teammate and I, out on our deck, our custom at that time of the year, late spring. We started a fire crackling in the chiminea (our outdoor fireplace) as it wasn't yet summer warmth.

Then I made my first mistake. So soon, so quickly. I said that Dr. K would like to see us tomorrow. "Together?" Marty asked. He'd gone into the doctor's office the previous Wednesday with questions about why he was experiencing a challenge just hoisting a speaker at his last gig, why his guitar was ponderous after a night of playing, why those muscles had been twitching oddly in his upper arm in the past while. For some time he'd struggled to play the more challenging gypsy jazz numbers he so loved. Thought it was arthritis in his hands.

He'd had tests. Short days ago. The import of a doctor phoning on a Sunday hung over us.

"He wants to see both of us tomorrow?" he asked to clarify.

"Tomorrow," I confirmed.

Did he look at the fire? Did he continue to look at me? Did he blink? Did he take a bite of food? I don't remember. But I do remember that then he said, "So why are you telling me now? Why didn't you wait until tomorrow?"

In that moment, with those words, I could feel some almost imperceptible shift.

I was the player running away with the ball. I've never been athletic. Anyone can tell you: Don't hand Alison the ball. She won't know what to do with it. But there I was, leaving him behind, streaking off to some other place. No one cheering. No sense of team. Maybe going in the wrong direction. I could be doing just that; I wouldn't know. No time to stop and ask for directions. No coach. No goalposts.

Black and White

MY EARLIEST MEMORY of television—like many Canadians—was Mr. Dressup, with his treehouse and his puppets, Casey and Finnegan. The television, a wooden box on legs, sat in the middle of our unfinished recreation room, concrete floor covered by a threadbare grandma-hand-me-down rug with raggedy fringe edge, and an ancient, fat couch that pushed my brother and I into L-shapes, legs sticking straight out on its deep cushions. We had Mr. Dressup and three other channels, one American from over the nearby border. Rabbit ears crowned the box.

We watched little. In fact, after *Mr. Dressup* we went without for almost a decade before we had another black-and-white, this time, a six-dollar purchase from the giant Sally Ann store in New Westminster, where my mother bought it on a whim at my older brother's urging. My older brother longed to see a hockey game, he said. He had all the convincing push of a television lawyer. So we had hockey. And *Little House on the Prairie*, and the odd ancient matinee. I remember only one really, and it was old even then: *The Pride of the Yankees – The Life of Lou Gehrig*. Its images filled my head, and haunted me in the way that television haunts those who are not inoculated against its visual power. I remember scenes of the beloved first baseman fumbling with a bat, and stumbling, and bits of his famous speech about being the luckiest man. My father must have explained to me what the diagnosis meant, because the film didn't go that far. I absorbed the information that the disease rendered the body inert, and one's brain became trapped inside one's body; that part stood out for me. Lou Gehrig's disease ended communication between brain and muscle. Eventually one could no longer move or speak, breathe or eat.

I knew that it moved quickly—though how quickly, I wasn't certain. I remembered thinking that this must be the worst way to die. I knew doctors had few answers, even yet, all these years later. It was not curable. I knew about Lou Gehrig's disease, about ALS, even though I could not have said what the A or L or S stood for.

More than thirty-five years later, our family doctor sat us in his office that Monday, June 1, 2015, and he said, "It could be MS, it could be ALS, it could be..." I didn't catch the third possibility. My teacher-brain thought, He's done it—he's used the sandwich approach. He's put the real diagnosis in between two pieces of white bread to try to make it go down.

ALS scared the shit out of me that 1970s Sunday afternoon in my parents' house on the second-hand black-and-white. It still did.

Where was Mr. Dressup now, when I needed him to draw a picture with those wax crayons of his, some picture that would help me make sense of this?

Amyotrophic.

Lateral.

Sclerosis.

4.

On Being
a Team

SOMETHING HAPPENED A little more than two years before that first of June.

After years of child-raising and devolving into that take-it-for-granted state that marriage frequently does in spite of best intentions, my spouse of almost twenty-five years and I fell in love.

Maybe it had something to do with friends' relationships doing otherwise. Or something of seeing the pain that middle-aged people can inflict on each other. Or maybe a curiosity about those around us who managed to hold on to each other and work through. Hard to say exactly what is the nature of such glue. Though it might be worth the analysis.

We spent time together as we hadn't in so long. Friends who knew us as people with rather separate lives—no, very separate lives—were surprised to see us together. We talked more, we laughed more, and we had to change our sheets frequently. We talked about growing old together as something to look forward to. We were a Team. An invincible team, I thought.

The Team: First, Marty. Short, five foot seven, quick on his feet, animated. Charismatic, even. Eyes like Buster Keaton. A musician who made most of his living from teaching guitar, occasionally bass or banjo, to local young people, or older people with ageing dreams, and groups of school kids. He earned the rest of his living with frequent gigs. He was well-loved in our community, and known for T-shirts with funny words or visuals, and quirky shoes.

Then there's me. Not so quick on my feet, even clumsy at times, and not so animated. Recovering introvert, in truth. Writer. Writing teacher. Mother of sons. Sister of brothers. Former tree-climber. With a thing for the warmth of fires crackling or hissing at my feet.

At that point in time when the youngest child is on the cusp of adulthood, marriages can go one way or the other. I felt fortunate ours went as it did. This second chance—that's what it seemed—taught me not to take a relationship for granted. It's so easy to get caught up in the dailies, and lost. I never wanted to be lost again. To remember what is important, people and connection above all, had become a mantra even before the first of June. I was ripe for testing, not that that's how I would have seen my life right then.

There are perks to being a Team, and the most sizeable is a sense of not being alone. As aloneness is the human state, if you have a good partner, you tend to feel you have escaped. There's a bit of wonder in that, at moments, maybe even something lacking humility; we'd done the impossible, beat the odds, the ugly, painful, and real odds.

I believed I knew a lot about ageing relationships.

Heroes—Just
For One Day

MY OLDEST SON spent many young hours as Batman. I made him a cardboard mask of cereal box, coated with thick black wax crayon. It's in the scrapbook now, the elastic to hold it in place over his face slack, and the cereal box card soft as flannel. A friend made him a cape with a cutaway scalloped edge, and I have photos and a strong mental image of him standing, red curls exploding around the mask, arms crossed solidly over his chest as preschoolers do, with grasped elbows, and with his bottom lip out slightly—enough to let you know not to give him any Trouble.

We do like to be heroes.

Days in, after diagnosis, I made a note in my journal of laundered bed sheets, and how it feels at the end of the day to slip into them—so much better. As if that would mend. Or put cape and mask on me.

This is what happens, with a diagnosis. Or at least, this is what happened with me: I heard the doctor speak, I went into some space of shock. We began to feel our way, and numbness set in, almost like being inside a hamster ball; I could see out, others could see in. Nothing could really touch me, though, and sounds were muted. I didn't eat much the first day, beyond the childhood comfort of tomato soup and a nibble of grilled cheese sandwich. But deep inside me a wee character had pulled on a cape, too, and her own little Batwoman mask, so tiny I didn't see her at first, but she began to grow.

She thought that things like clean sheets made a difference.

6.

Preliminary Diagnosis

WE CLUNG TO the word "preliminary" and the boys—told later—did so too. I also knew the prognosis; maybe Marty didn't know about that as much as I did. The blessing of shock kept the knowledge ever so slightly removed. That's what shock does. Lets the knowledge leak in just a bit at a time.

Later that afternoon, that very first Monday, I took Marty a cup of coffee in his teaching studio and found him staring at his computer. "It says three to four years," he said, wonderingly.

"I don't think you should do that," I said. "Don't research online. Just ask Dr. K your questions. Or I can look up stuff."

He closed the page, took the coffee. Said he would prepare for his afternoon of guitar students and that I should go do what I had planned. He stood and we hugged.

"We don't know yet," I reminded him. "Not for sure."

THE MORNING AFTER the appointment with Dr. K, while we lay in bed, I put my hand on Marty's bicep and felt the fasciculations of the muscles—twitching and pulsing, just as I'd felt for the past couple of months. I pulled my hand away, repulsed. Felt badly. Wrapped an arm around his midriff instead. It occurred to me then that we were still us. Even as my mind struggled with the rest.

The F. Scott Fitzgerald quote came to mind: "The test of a first-rate intelligence is the ability to hold two opposed ideas in mind at the same time and still retain the ability to function."

That was my truth at the moment. Or at least, the piece about trying to hold on to two opposed ideas, though I was not certain what the two ideas were.

The sentence that follows in the Fitzgerald quote: "One should, for example, be able to see that things are hopeless and yet be determined to make them otherwise."

What was otherwise? Hope? Acceptance? Yes, these two could push at each other.

Little Batwoman grew.

I KNEW—REALLY—FROM THE moment the doctor said ALS that we were facing terminal. After that, it was confirmation, and coming to terms. It can take a long time to come to terms with terminal.

7.

Old Vows

THE DAY AFTER that Marty awoke with a sob. The feral sound made something in my gut curl. It made my thoughts scatter, and I tried to retrieve them but didn't know how to do that. I wrapped an arm around him, but he loosened my hold and went to shower, and I lay in bed thinking that we were not even forty-eight hours in, and already I couldn't think what came next, what to do next. All that came to mind: *This is the shittiest thing ever.*

He came out of the bathroom and dressed. Sat on the edge of the bed and said he was certain he did indeed have ALS. Dr. K said that being overly emotional was a marker, maybe *the* marker, for the disease. Emotional lability, a result of frontal lobe dysfunction. Unlike most GPs, our doctor had had more than one previous patient with this disease.

I remembered then that when Marty returned in February, from a trip to Mexico with his brother and cousin, he was unsettled by his own tears at the airport. At the time we talked about how perhaps it was ageing and something of recognizing what others mean to us. But I recalled how this apparent betrayal of his emotions had shaken him. He didn't like to be openly emotional.

Then, before leaving the bedroom, he said he didn't want to be a burden. I said that wouldn't happen. I meant it. I couldn't imagine that he would be a burden. Or if he became such, the work involved wouldn't feel burdensome. It would simply be. It would be part of choosing to spend lives together. It would be the "in sickness" part of the vows, though I honestly couldn't recall what our Unitarian vows had been; it didn't matter. My understanding of vowing to spend lives together included this. Simultaneously, I was grateful that we'd come to mean more to each other in the last two years. The time of falling back into love, remembering where we'd come from—indeed, feeling it to have been something it never was even in younger years—all those months had been building strength for this.

After he left the bedroom to go to his studio downstairs, I lay immersed in thoughts about "burden." And came to the conclusion that while I didn't know how to navigate this path yet, I would figure it out. This could be the opportunity to show how much I loved him and what he meant to me. I felt a sense of relief when my mind found this as an answer, and fastened my being around that word "opportunity." Perhaps hope could win over numbness.

When I got downstairs, he wasn't yet working in his studio; the vacuum roared in the living room. He did not vacuum on a regular basis. But when he was anxious he would, or he would sweep or dust.

Usually the anxious cleaning bothered me. He would do some furious dusting before our annual Christmas music party, while I finalized food, and food always seemed so much more significant than dust that it would leave me feeling agitated. Or the act of sweeping while his sister was dying, and I tried my best to convince him to buy a plane ticket to Regina to be with her. He'd swept the entire deck, an otherwise useless task, without speaking a word.

But that day, two days after the preliminary diagnosis, I shut up and let him vacuum. Maybe after he turned it off, set it down, left to work, I'd take it up myself and do it all again.

Later, going grocery shopping, I cried backing out of the driveway. Somehow leaving my home, even for an hour, seemed not right. For one, it was so ordinary; how could we do the ordinary? It was also a leaving. Everything felt to be a leaving. Everything felt to be extra-ordinary.

Driving to the store, I saw an old couple, greyed, holding hands as they walked the sidewalk. I'd had grey hair already for years myself, but Marty's hair was still a shade of ginger, and I realized I'd been looking forward to seeing if he would age as his father had, with a gently retreating hairline. Indeed, I *was* looking forward to Future. To Growing Old Together. To being sixty-four and will you still love me, and all. Being sixty-four was still more than a decade away for me. Marty was fifty-seven.

Groceries in the backseat an hour later, and I spotted the smoke shop. In the past eight or nine months, I'd nagged about too much drinking, now realizing this had not been about alcohol amounts but about the neurological response to his usual two post-golf-game beers. All the hours I'd worried about his smoking over the years. I'd never been too good at nagging, and the worry had cost me.

I went into the smoke shop and bought a cigar that cost about as much as steak dinner for two. Wished I'd done this for Christmas years ago. He did like a cigar with those two beers.

I went home, packed things into the fridge. How normal it felt. And did not feel.

Pulled on yoga pants—let's keep some normal going—prepped to go to class.

Marty came into the kitchen to refill coffee, and we hugged, an almost normalizing hug before I went to the leisure centre. I worked to keep a light tone to my voice; was that the right thing to do?

At the end of yoga class, lying in savasana, I cried.

A portrait of a day. An early day in a new life.

WHEN I SAW our doctor, one-on-one that first week, to ask questions I didn't want Marty to hear, there was a moment when he said his name—"Marty"—and I heard it almost as the first time someone said "your son" to me after the birth of our first child: a moment of recognition of connection. A moment of a type of pride. Not unhealthy pride. How to explain such a moment, how to explain feeling tears over simply hearing a name.

8.

The Search Thing

THAT FIRST WEEK was in slow motion. Then it sped up.

The Search Thing. "Don't go on the Internet," said Dr. K. He didn't say the word "terminal," but it had its hold over us.

Someone mentioned Stephen Hawking: "He's lived with this for *years*." Right! I'd forgotten that ALS was his diagnosis. The Internet became hard to resist.

I wanted positives and things I could *do*. Because it was horrific not being able to do anything. Especially if one has an inner nascent—and carping—Batwoman.

Online, I learned about drugs, exercise, and food—modern salvation.

The only drug for this disease at that time, riluzole, was not particularly useful, from all reports. It might extend life by weeks or a couple of months, but the time tacked on to the end of the path, and in no way appeared to extend the outset. Even early on, this did not seem desirable.

Exercise would not improve well-being. In fact, weight-resistance and running were off the table—though it did seem that it would be good to golf, to walk and breathe in the green outdoors. But anything that would bring on any level of exhaustion was to be avoided. The disease is one of constant sense of fatigue. Once tired, there is no "recovery."

The short list of muscles unaffected by this disease included bladder, bowels, heart, intestines, sex organs. All was not lost. And eyes were on the list. I'd always thought I could read Marty's eyes, that they said enough.

As for food. Try not to lose weight. Once one lost 10 percent of body mass, there was a quick decline in health, said an article I stumbled over. So—rich meals, snacks, smoothies, protein shakes.

I went grocery shopping again, this time with a lighter step.

We celebrated my findings and my sense of There-Is-Something-I-Can-Do by having a full-on roast chicken dinner, organic of course, with brown rice stuffing, mashed potatoes, Yorkshire puddings, gravy, and multiple vegetables. I hummed while I worked, and felt almost giddy. I couldn't squelch the feeling of hope.

In the middle of the night, I awoke. Marty spooned around me, and I could feel what seemed to be every muscle in his body twitching, jumping, restless. I'd thought it was only in his biceps. How had it come to this? How had I not noticed before? Or was it this sudden?

After more research on Hawking, I discovered he had the rarer form of juvenile ALS, with which one can live an average lifespan, albeit not a normal life.

Roast chicken, Batwoman, and the Internet.

9.

What About the Boys?

What to tell the boys. When
to tell. *Why*
to tell… maybe it is
a nightmare, and we are going to
awaken
and it won't be necessary
to say anything
Our boys—23, 19, 16
Cleve, Ole, Emmett. Young men
on the edge

How are we going to get through? If
I can't even tell them
what is happening now, how
are we going to get through?

10.

A Good Question

I HAD TO head into town for a meeting with my writing partner of many years, Gayle. I thought about not going. But Marty was golfing, my story had been written, and I had comments prepared for the piece she'd shared with me. And we were busy pretending it might be something else. Or nothing. It seemed right to let the pretending stretch into other areas of our lives. So Marty continued to teach students, and I kept such appointments.

I drove into the city. Coming out of a gas station, to my right a car almost drove into me, and I found myself screaming in anger at the driver. "You can't kill me!" He couldn't. I couldn't die. Because that would make my children orphans, and they needed me. "I have too much to do! You can't kill me!" His car disappeared down the road, and I sat, shaking, worn out from screaming, and the thought, and the truth of the thought.

I drove on to Gayle's, feeling not quite in my body. Once there, I realized I didn't know how or what to tell her. We offered our writing feedback to each other, as usual. Work is always the thread that we can hold on to until we can't.

Gayle and I had worked together for more than two decades. After our work, I told her.

We cried. She smoked a cigarette. I enjoyed her smoking a cigarette.

She asked me, "How much time do you spend wishing things weren't what they are?"

The question stopped me. I tried to measure. Bits of my life came to mind. Bits I resisted. Bits I welcomed. What did I push back against? What did I allow to wash over me, or flow around?

How much time did I spend wishing things weren't what they were?

"Not much," I answered. "Not usually, anyway."

The question stayed with me through the months. It became a line to sort—some things on one side of it, and some on the other. Then I would move thoughts from one to the other. I thought about the question enough that it would enter my mind without consciously thinking about it, habitually. Usefully. It kept me on a path, checked me at times.

I sent her an email the following day. Thank you for being a good friend, for listening and looking right at me. I know there are going to be people in my life who, when I tell them this, I'll feel energy draining out of me. But then there is someone like you, and I feel energy coming in.

Fig Leaves

I STEPPED OUTSIDE, taken by the shininess of the leaves of my fig tree. The tree, seven years old, as wide as tall, swallowed an entire corner of the yard, and the leaves were huge and bright yellowy green. A sunny, happy colour. In August the fruit would be heavy, tumescent, hidden behind those leaves, yet soaking sun into the pink sweetness. Too sweet, really.

In the afternoon, I stepped outside again. Marty was getting a CAT scan; this is how ALS is diagnosed—by a process of eliminating other possibilities. I felt short of breath, and a wave of claustrophobia. Not my usual state, though I'd long witnessed my mother succumbing to this. But this claustrophobia felt to have something of a desire to escape; perhaps all claustrophobia is this. I had a sudden curious desire to take my short nails to my skin and tear it off. The feeling did not last long and—following my instinct to be out of doors—once outside I breathed slower, more fully, and the skin-scrape urge passed. (I had yet to know the force of this urge.) But I noticed, as I looked into the yard from my deck, that the leaves of the fig tree were no longer their happy green. Even though the sun shone bright as ever for the day, maybe more so, the leaves were dulled, their green a flat shade.

It wasn't the leaves, I realized, stunned; it was me. How did that work? Was the physical so connected to the emotional that my eyes saw differently?

In the evening, dusk on the deck, I spotted bats whooshing flappity-flap overhead for the first time in three years. I was inordinately happy to see them. Days of ups and downs. These were just the early days; up and down became a pattern. A new normal.

First Weekend

WE WENT TO a local musical performance, a friend, Mike G, who also played guitar. Marty chose seats on the far edge, close to the back, as if preparing for flight. Such an odd choice for him. And yes, we did leave early, he leading the way with no explanation. He just got up and started to walk out, and I followed. The place was a seniors' recreation centre, with a lovely small stage, and large window overlooking a garden. Although I'd walked through the garden before, I'd never stopped there, and that evening I sat on a bench we found, with the familiar stranger I called husband. It's always an odd thing, to find a new corner in a town you've lived in for decades; the whole was in keeping with the week we'd just lived, and even with that moment.

Couldn't remember ever leaving a musical event so early, let alone a friend's performance. We sat just outside the doorway. Part of me dreaded our friend or his spouse coming outside on a break, seeing us, and asking the innocent, "How are you?" Behind that would be *Why have you left early?*

We sat in silence for a bit, then talked. I found myself puzzling through, aloud. Perhaps not the best plan, as everything

I said seemed not to come out as I'd intended. I began to talk about how we were two sides of the same coin; this was how I'd been seeing us over the days of this week, as my thoughts hovered. But as soon as I said this aloud, muttered something about being back to back, so close, yet going in utterly opposite directions, Marty either did not want to get my intended meaning, or had nothing to say about it. He just looked at me blankly. I stopped mid-sentence. We talked about going home instead. "Let's make a fire on the deck," I suggested. I needed to keep it light. Yet be ready for when it might change. And keep my thoughts to myself as I worked my way through them.

Some years before, we'd added a large deck to the side of the house, with a high roof over half of it, which made it useable through many months in our rainy climate. Even though the local municipality had a bylaw about open fires, we had a metal-screened outdoor fireplace, a chiminea. My father had built us a sizeable tiled hearth on wheels, to go underneath and catch sparks. When the rain came, we would pull the chiminea under the roof, and continue even into the fall. It was our favourite place. As friends rushed to their cabins for the weekend, we liked to joke about our far-away recreation spot. The deck, about eighteen inches off the ground, did not require a railing, and so we'd designed it leaving the support posts high, and had put large rings in them, and I could snap on a hammock in a moment, for afternoon reading, or evening fireside.

That Friday night we built a fire, poured wine, put feet up.

I asked Marty what he'd like to do this summer. I thought we should go and visit family. But he said he wanted to do three things: play golf with friends; have his summer Rock

School camp with his music students; and this, sit by the fire in the evening. In other words, a normal summer, though even this seemed, to me at least, to require hero effort.

"I don't want to be that guy," he said, toward the end of the conversation, after a short period of silence.

"What guy?" I said.

"In that movie we saw."

I had to think.

"The one your workmate wrote."

The Sue Rodriguez story. "That was a woman."

He appeared not to have heard me. "The one who blinked his eyes to say yes and no. I don't want to do that."

"I don't think we can really think about that," I said. "That's a long time from now." My thoughts: I had to learn about these things, and pull together some ideas and knowledge. Quickly.

Then: "What's going to become of me?" he asked, for the first time. He would ask this at several points in the months to come. This time, after thinking, I said, "We'll take care of you," and that seemed to satisfy him. For the moment.

One and then another of our sons joined us. We were glad for the distraction. One took photos. The photos revealed nothing; masks were in place to protect the boys.

After the fire died down, I talked Marty into making love. I remember hoping it would take us someplace else. I remember that it was just sad.

13.

Team Intact—
Momentarily

TEN DAYS AFTER diagnosis, and holding on—somewhat—
while hunting for stove cleaner, I found a leak in the kitchen
sink plumbing. The garbage pail sat in slurpy bubbles on the
soaked plywood floor of the cupboard. And I lost it. I began
to mutter, curse, louder and louder again. Marty heard and
came, and even as he did, my brain began to take over and
rationalize. After all, the tap had been dripping for a while
now. What did I expect?

I held the phone flashlight, and he tightened the connection, checked the other side, then stood and did his Mr. Fixit
pose. We laughed and hugged. The moment was light and
good, and I wanted it to stretch as long as it could. There
would always be time to feel sad and weird. At that moment,
light was good. Was some part of each of us holding on to
hope? That somehow Dr. K had made a mistake? Or that the
tests would hold a surprise?

Later that day, Marty let me know he appreciated this. "I
like it when you are positive." Yet I'd been wondering if my
trying to keep it light might not indicate that I seemed not
to care as much as I did.

Stay with the light...

14.

Dream

In the morning I awake from a dream. I don't often
recall dreams
They usually disappear to some deep place
But in this one, vivid, I knock on an unfamiliar door. It
doesn't feel unknown to me though. My grandpa, gone for
close to twenty years
stands in the open doorway
with the shadow of facial hair on his sunned face, his
steel grey curls thick
and sticking up, always

He doesn't say a word, but there are tears in his eyes
We look at each other for a long time, it feels
Then I wake up
His face, those tears, stays with me throughout the day

15.

Into June

BEFORE WE TOLD the boys anything, we had to go to Marty's mother's house in Saskatchewan to pack up her home of decades and move her into a seniors' residence. We'd made plans for this and purchased plane tickets months before. We decided we would tell the boys about their father after we returned home. I did not want to tell them beforehand, and then leave them alone while they were absorbing what this might mean. We also decided to tell Marty's brother and sister before we left. His mom was in some state of senility, and we decided she didn't need to know at all at that point. It would be too much along with losing her home.

A full set of nieces and nephews—five in all, half-orphaned when Marty's sister passed away six years before—we decided we wouldn't tell them, either. Again, it would be too much, with having lost their mom. But mostly it would also be too much for Marty, with the emotional mayhem of ALS.

He was a bit of a mess in this really. As much as I hoped I could manage my own emotional mess, his had the added impact of being neurological.

Less than two weeks in and it was hard to keep secrets, yet hard to share and feel people leaning on me. At that point, it wasn't so much something I could articulate as it was an awareness of Things To Avoid.

Off we flew, to the prairie.

What I remember from that week is now just a series of images:

Looking at the double bed where my mother-in-law had slept for years, alone since 1994. One side of the bed was substantially lower than the other; she must never have moved to the middle. Is that what widows did? Some part of me took mental notes and tried not to feel terrified. Not for the first time, I was grateful to be a writer. I could make use of my writing process, to sit with ideas, with the immediate, with possibilities, and with looming realities. Even as another part of me wanted not to put words to anything, and another part of me wanted to run away. Or just be someone else. Not for the first or last time I wondered, *Is this my life?* Had I blundered into someone else's?

We pulled the bed away from the wall, and found dust thick as velvet. The smell in the room was the sour smell of an old woman. Correction: an old woman who never seemed comfortable with the physical act of love. A lonely room, an alone woman. Age just covered it, wrapped it, sorrowed it.

Another image: The bin at the foot of the driveway, filling with the stuff of Home of decades. That mattress, the bedstead, ancient fruitcakes (she wanted to know where they'd gone. *Where?!*) and food tins that would thrill a film props decorator. Even a box of Toni hair permanent—the set decorator would swoon!

Her oatmeal got tossed in with a satisfying clunk.

At the close of the day, my mother-in-law wanted that, her oatmeal in its cylindrical cardboard. Where was it?

We couldn't leave the house until we promised to replace it. Would mealy-wormed oatmeal matter if she knew that she was in the process of losing the second of four children? The oatmeal might matter to her—senility had her. Memories and what-is-important comes and goes. Oatmeal was security.

Another image: My niece, talking at some point in those Saskatchewan days, of losing her mother. (Every time I see the prairie, I am transported in time to our beginnings as a family. Summer weeks at the cabin. The lake with the drone of bagpipes over it on a Sunday aft, the furtive love-making that happens at family gatherings, with so many ears around.) Again, some part of me took note as my niece spoke of her young knowledge of death. I needed to know this, I needed to anticipate my sons' needs. Even though they were on the cusp of adulthood—our oldest had recently bought a condo, and would be moving in six weeks—at least, that had been the plan—I expected this would re-route their paths to some degree. Hard to say how. But the mother part of me busied herself in that corner of my mind. The mother's mind is like a work room with stations, punching timecards for each, or is remiss. This mind was melding with the caregiving mind.

So when my niece spoke of how her family seemed to disintegrate after the fact, I listened. I didn't want to lose my boys too. The thought took away my breath.

I spent a full morning with my sister-in-law packing up her mother's house, and returned to Marty at his brother's home, napping, watching golf on TV. He said he'd missed me for those few hours.

The question occurred to both of us: Would the nieces notice those naps? Already, napping was necessary. So quickly. As if once the diagnosis had been acknowledged— or at least what we were handed so far—the symptoms could lurch from sleep to a stand and take off.

Thinking about how, not long ago, we were a couple with evening after evening spent apart. Sometimes days passed with few words between us. Now, I was down the street for a few hours, and he missed me. What could life ask of us not to take another for granted?

Before we left to return home, I wrote to a friend, Tammy, who also had three sons, the ages of our boys, who had lost their father. I wrote to ask if she would share with me how they'd told their boys that their father was so ill. Maybe there was some way to say this that softened, or at least made the cut clean. (What healed more easily, I tried to remember from the book about birthing that I read so long ago, a clean cut or a natural tear?) The need to tell my children their father was dying was so strong. I tried to tell myself he was ill—that was all they needed to know. But I knew it was more than that. The need was a desperate push, a feeling that wouldn't let me go until they knew. I wished that someone could tell me how to do it, and how it would go, and how they would be after the telling. How I would be.

I didn't let Marty know that I was thinking it'd be best to tell them on Saturday, the day after we returned home. The alternative, Sunday, was Father's Day. There was a fragility to him, and an urge in me to protect. If I left such things to last minute, there was less time to experience pain. I was learning.

On the flight home, we were unexpectedly given seats five rows apart for the first leg of the trip, as far as Calgary. There was panic on my husband's face, a look I'd never seen before. I suspected this would not be the first time for this facial expression. I had to reassure him that after Calgary we'd have adjoining seats. He looked back at me, and seemed lost making his way farther down the aisle. I fought the feeling of having just dropped off a child at kindergarten for the first time. We were all grownups here. Or maybe it was me who was dropped off. Watching the back of someone, walking away.

Will you be back at the end of the day? That was what the child wanted to know. How had this man become a child again? How had I become... what? How had this gotten *here* so quickly?

When I thought about the past months, almost the past year, there had been symptoms. The times I'd thought Marty had had more than two beers, when he swore that was all, even as he mumbled a bit and dragged his feet; the time he stumbled over the hearth; and, oddly, the way he would move his head, and his eyes took a split second to follow. It made me wonder how long he had been experiencing symptoms. And why he'd said nothing.

"You're very observant," said the neurologist, when I mentioned the bit about his eyes and the split second.

But I'd missed so much.

16.

Tammy Says

You'll plan one hundred ways to tell them and in the
end
it'll blurt out in some way
unplanned
Also, she says
(when I tell her my fears)
you'll understand Marty when he speaks
(how does she know this?)
Later—she means *after*—all you'll remember
are the good parts

And, she says
never turn down any offer of help

17.

How to Tell the Children

IT CAME DOWN to Father's Day. It had to be. Or wait several more days, which I didn't want to do. Afterward, toward the end of the day, our oldest son Cleve said that it was a good day to let them know because the day came to mean more. I was aghast that those words came out of his mouth, but felt some rush of strange gratefulness, too. That somehow this man-child of twenty-three could see this and thought to say it.

I planned a hundred possible ways for the telling to roll out, but in the end, I was in tears, choking out something—I don't remember exactly what—but in the end, the message got out even if the words didn't. Cleve's first words were, "Can we get it?" Ole asked, "How long?" Emmett, the youngest, began to cry last.

The night before, discussing this by the fire, Marty had asked me not to name the illness, and just to let them know something of what it might mean. We tried to work around that, but in the end, Marty did end up saying "ALS" when one of them asked for the name. And then I explained a bit of what that meant. The Ice Bucket Challenge had been just the summer before, the national ALS fundraising event, and Ole had enthusiastically taken part, so he had some idea. We let them know that although Dr. K thought he knew the diagnosis, and their dad was exhibiting symptoms, conclusive tests had not yet been done.

Marty did the cooking—omelettes in the porcelain frypan—even though he was convinced no one would eat. But Ole, athletic son, dug in and ate, which was good because then we both felt useful—me, because I cut up everything to create the "cooking show" scenario, grateful, grateful for habit and ritual, and Marty felt necessary, too. The others poked at their food, ate less, but did eat. As would be true in the months to come, each son handled the process much as they lived life. I was learning that dying and death does not fundamentally change people.

We walked about, first in stunned silence and then stunned speaking, before Marty went to play a Father's Day round of golf—golf can be stunned too—and then we all met for dinner at the golf course, a Father's Day buffet, and wondered how we'd pulled off this day. Someone came by and responded to our request to take photos of us at the table, not realizing what exactly he was documenting. How did we smile?

Maybe with the relief of having done the telling. That urge to tell my children, the urge that had filleted my gut, I wrapped in duct tape and stuffed into the back of the closet. For the time, at least.

I knew that they were holding on to the thought that not all the testing had been done. That maybe, somehow, the results would read differently to a specialist. We were all hoping. There were now more people holding on to hope.

White Rock Guitar

THERE WAS A guitarist performing a half-hour drive away in the neighbouring town of White Rock. I can't remember the name of the artist. It was the last day of June, the last day of the worst month of my life. Some of Marty's guitar students would be at the show, and musician friends.

Summer evenings are a gift, with the warmth, the sweater-free of it, the light shoes. I usually took mine off, if I was the passenger in the car or the mom sitting at a ballgame. I love the feeling of bare feet.

Marty climbed into the Corolla. Growing up in Saskatchewan, he could drive anything. He could drive at age twelve, in heavy snow, hail, pulling donuts on ice, whatever. He had perfect control of any vehicle. He'd taught our boys to drive, and me to drive standard.

We left Ladner, and set out on the highway. Marty took the quickest route, he always did. I would choose the scenic, the backroads, or sometimes the more familiar way. He prided himself on finding shortcuts and quick routes—paths others miss. He drove fast. He tailgated, always confident that he'd manage to brake in time. Fair enough, I suppose, after a lifetime of no accidents. Always observant, and he could see with the eyes of a fly, peripheral vision switched on, foot ready.

We approached a section of highway, busy with over-passes and exits, and ahead of us cars had their brake lights red. Had Marty noticed? He wasn't slowing, even though he said something about traffic. I was loath to point this out to him, as he never did *not* notice, and if I pulled his attention to something he could quickly become annoyed with me. He knew, he'd say, and had said, many times. He always knew. But maybe not that time. The other cars had slowed, even stopped, and he was still full on. Last minute, I called out, "Marty—they're stopped!"

He turned the wheel, a split-second decision, and took us between the left lane cars and the concrete median. Our car met the median, with the sound of crush, but out my window drivers' surprised faces flashed by.

Then we stopped. We're all right, I thought. We haven't hit anyone. We are not hurt. It could have been bad, very bad. If I hadn't called out.

Marty said something about how this happened because he was distracted by why the people in the turn lane were stopped. But we were in the left-hand lane, with no reason to be thinking about the exit of traffic. He was lying, and he knew I knew it.

Traffic slowly moved ahead, and we pulled into the lane when it cleared, and took our place. I still felt as if I couldn't breathe. I was thinking about our boys, about how their dad was dying, and about how they needed me to be here. How there was *there* and there was *here*. How we couldn't both go. We drove in silence for long minutes, and then softly he said, "I'm sorry, honey." He reached out and took my hand, which was rare. The word *sorry* was filled with something raw and real, probably the most sincere apology I'd ever had from him, and I absorbed what it might mean. More than a near miss. We didn't speak again until we were off the highway. He held back from the other cars.

White Rock, a beach town with hilly streets pushing up from the water, had old-style angle parking. Last time we were in this town it was for our twenty-fifth anniversary stay-home vacation and we had a pint, and Marty took a photo of me. When I'm happy, I look good. Photos of me looking good are only from the last few of our years together; it took me that long to know happy.

That June evening, we parked as if our lives depended on it. Now we did many simple daily things as if this was so. Maybe it was. We checked the side of the car, surprised to find only the lightest of scraping—it had sounded like so much more. We crossed the street.

We saw familiar faces as we approached the theatre. Our neighbours, Marty's former student and father. More familiar faces even, and I was aware that the person with me didn't really want to be seen tonight. Most unusual for him. We ducked through the doorway, and sat about two-thirds of the way from the front and not on aisle seats. All so different from how we usually did things. Was he finding new footing, new ways to be in the world? There was no conviviality. We left early, as the last song started. True, Marty always left bigger concerts at that point, but not in the more intimate settings such as this, when he'd linger, find someone to go for a beer, and talk afterward to compare thoughts about the performance.

We ducked out—yes, the sense of "ducking"—heads down, moving quickly, as quickly as we could, though already we were slowed by him. As we neared the car, he said he'd drive... if I trusted him. I said okay, just please leave a lot of space. Enough to buy time. He did. We were quiet on the way home, too. A thick quietness that had nothing of the gift of a summer evening.

Team 2

OUR MAILBOX WAS large and wooden. There might be a moth hiding in it, a moth that would come flapping out. There were often pieces of garden equipment or tools tucked in quickly after some chore, and forgotten. I never knew what I'd find in there in addition to pieces of mail.

I pulled out a letter, return address Vancouver General Hospital, addressed to Mr. Martin H____. Not thinking— tired from no sleep—I handed it to him in his studio as he waited for a student to show up.

He opened it. It was only to confirm an appointment. But it threw off his morning, his day even. It reminded him. It reminded me. I should have kept it to myself.

I so wanted to keep the team together. To play centre as needed, and goalie, and cheerleader. Mixing my sports and metaphors. Didn't matter. I just wanted the team.

But I couldn't share anymore. In the name of protection, I couldn't. I had to remember to keep things to myself.

20.

Snapshots

SOME TIMES STAND out in our minds. Thinking about them, reviewing them, becomes something like the olden days when we'd slowly make our way through an album of photographs—sticky paper and plastic in the '70s, and black paper and shiny photo corners before then.

How did life come to be in snapshots? Maybe we don't want the progression of film. Maybe in a snapshot—even a mental one—we can stop time for just a spell before moving on to the next. Even a series of snapshots can have a reassuring quality of static. We don't have to move on; we can always close the album.

July 15 was a series of snapshots. Postcards. *Wish I wasn't here.*

The series began with a message. *I'm doing second loop,* texted Marty as I checked my phone after my flamenco class. Translation: Round 2 of golf, then having a beer. So it was later when I went to pick him up from the golf course. It was dusk, and the sky had that luminous indigo teal to it, colour that always pulls me back to being a preschooler, and working on a Disney big-piece puzzle with my mom. That was when I became acquainted with gradations of teal (prior to the '80s and my hair colour). It's a time of day that—perhaps because of that memory—relaxes me. At times, in spite of myself.

But before I could get out of the car at the club, I saw two figures emerge, and one had an arm around another, a small other, my husband. He was in tears, clutching his vapourizer (always trying to stop smoking, at times successful, other times not), dragging his feet. I could see immediately that he was quite drunk. Not that that took much. That was snapshot number one. Marty, clutching, holding on physically, and emotionally in bits.

He had to be helped into the car by Cory, a golf course employee and friend. Cory slipped the vapourizer into the pocket of the car door, and gave me a deep look before gently closing the door.

Marty leaned back for a moment, and cried. Then we hugged.

Snapshot number two: To my left, driving home, the sun setting. "Everyone is so nice to me," Marty marvelled. "People love you," I said.

"I can't think of words I want to say," he admitted. "I know them, but they don't come out."

That scared me.

"And really, my hands haven't worked for a long time."

I didn't ask him why he hadn't told me. He was giving voice to the things that scared him and had been scaring him, and I didn't want to say anything that might stop this. I wanted him to feel safe telling me.

Snapshot number three. As we arrived home, Cleve and Ole were both pulling into driveway, too, a veritable family traffic jam, a train to the front door. Marty stumbled on the step, but didn't fall. Not that time.

Snapshot number four. Minutes later, sitting on the back deck, Ole amused his dad with a story of a ridiculously big club for a golf contest, and Marty was laughing so hard. That lability of ALS. But good to see him laughing, yes.

Later, the sudden exhaustion of bedtime—Marty waited for that exhaustion, stayed up for it, so he wouldn't have to lie awake in bed. He'd be falling-down tired when he put in his earbuds for the night, and fell asleep to his podcast soundtrack. Beside him, I heard the peripheral whine, and was wide awake. Time passed. That was not a snapshot. That was a feeling, deep inside me. It was about two in the morning, and I needed to move. I knew Emmett would still be awake.

I pulled on a summer dress in the dark and found my sweater from Ole—how I loved that sweater, the one I thought I'd lost on an airplane the previous summer, taking him to school in Oklahoma, and I was so sad. Was that just a year before? What a thing to be sad about—the loss of a garment. Yet *that* thought made me sad. Someday could I be sad about normal-sad things? We could have travelled a bit farther when we were in Oklahoma, to see my friend in Austin. *We should have done a lot of things.*

I went downstairs, where I found Emmett, gamer, gaming into the small hours, as he loved to do. So strange to know that our home was connected with kids as far away as the UK at this time of night.

The words "Do you want to go on a walk with me?" were hardly out of my mouth and he was up from his chair without a word to Nigel on the other side of the Atlantic.

But before we left, standing by the heavy wooden table (snapshot number five), he asked, "Has it been confirmed?"

I realized he believed my sleeplessness, my request for a walk, had a Reason. I realized my children were still waiting for official confirmation. And were still hopeful. I realized how much I loathed being the person whose job it was to quash those hopes. Even though I knew better, I still had my own.

I had to say, "No, it hasn't been officially confirmed."

Does my memory hold? Did I wait until we set off down 52nd Avenue to say, "We do know what it is, though." Was there a bit of a question mark in that, asking him if he knew? He nodded, whether at the table, or gusting along the street. That's the problem with a snapshot, you can't see a nod. Like a telephone, and no visual.

Outside, indigo and teal were long gone. It was dark, and summer wind made the sky clear and bright. We both love to walk and set a fast pace.

He commented on the wind and what a nice night it was. I spoke my thought about how everyone now said, "Life is cruel," but the planet was still so beautiful. That thought came into my head almost every day. It pushed, it juxtaposed with the ugly. I needed the juxtaposition, the reminder.

We trudged for over an hour. We talked about how he saw our lives now. He said he felt he needed to keep Dad cheery.

I told him how I love all my boys. He wrapped an arm around me and told me I'd always been a great mom. That was nice of him to offer, and I stopped myself from saying something facetious about the "always" bit. We moved on from talk of his dad to random subjects, even as something hung over us. We walked all the way down to 45th Avenue, and turned the corner; there was one friend's home, and then another. I hadn't told them yet. I had seen one of these friends, John D, at the bank just a few days before, and I couldn't bring myself to say anything. I'd already talked to two people that day, and hit my limit.

We saw lights on in some homes, television light in some, warm lamp light in others. Snapshot six.

We made our way back home, wind pushing at us, and Emmett returned to his game.

In the dark, in our room, with Marty breathing, with podcast whining, I stripped off my outdoor clothes and climbed into bed. I suddenly knew that there would be a time when I wouldn't be able to leave at night and just go for a walk. I tried not to think ahead. The night was fresh, the wind was good. It cleared cobwebs, as my mother would say.

Snapshot: a lot of cobwebs in corners.

Preliminary Diagnosis

AMYOTROPHIC LATERAL SCLEROSIS is pronounced with a long A. It took me a while to know how to say it; these are not words you hear. It took me longer to realize that in the UK it is called MND, or Motor Neuron Disease, and that led me to a handbook published in Oxford. It became my real source of information, far more so than the local Vancouver ALS Clinic which, in spite of their best efforts, was a bleak place located in the windowless basement of the GF Strong Clinic Rehabilitation Centre building—a building Soviet Union in appearance. Why the basement for this disease? was a question in my mind every time we went there, and more often. The walls had the ubiquitous nature murals, a sad attempt to make it what it could not be. What does it take from one's soul to work with the dying? What kind of person can transform that? Can it *feed* one's soul?

Some parts of the Clinic Team were more useful and involved than others. I could see how, in the slower iterations of the disease, each would have a greater responsibility. But we steam-rolled through the stages, and the experts took walk-on roles. I could see their consternation over the progression of Marty's ALS. I believe they tried not to let this show, but it did. Their attempts not to show revealed humanity. But they never told me the things that I learned from that handbook: that the rate of progression was equal to rate of onset (and the onset had been so quick). Or that smaller people (Marty weighed 140 pounds) just don't live as long. Certain things were easier to read than to hear. My idea—from all those years before, seeing the Lou Gehrig movie—that the ALS mind is a clear one, was squelched by that book. Only 20 percent of people with ALS have a clear mind. Five percent have outright dementia. Three-quarters of people with the disease are somewhere between. Marty's cognitive fog seemed to be in the middle. Once, trying to decide whether or not to even consider chelation therapy— suggested by a golf partner—he was in tears, because he couldn't come up with yes or no. But he also couldn't decide what shoes to wear.

The occupational therapist was helpful, both in person and by email. When I wrote to ask her about the changes we would have to make to the downstairs bathroom so that Marty could stay at home, she sent photographs, with suggestions and dimensions for a chair to be access-ible and useful in the shower. In our meetings, she was able to demonstrate products that could make the difference between holding an eating utensil and not—pipes of con-densed foam to wrap around spoon or fork—and she showed me pictures of specialized knives that could enable one to cut food for weeks after a normal table-knife had been set aside. (I ordered one as soon as we arrived home from our first meeting.) This information was useful. Fine motor skills quickly became difficult. We were grateful for extensions of weeks, days, even hours, as the disease moved on.

EVEN THOUGH OUR doctor knew it was ALS, and we knew, too, really, there were still the formalities of neurologists having their looks and says.

The first neurologist we saw poked Marty with needles, apologized for the poking, and said that she had had one patient in the past who had exhibited all the symptoms of ALS, and sometime later they mysteriously disappeared. I wasn't certain whether that was a good thing to hear or not. It certainly played with the hope and acceptance possibilities.

So the summer held appointments, first at Vancouver General, then at the Clinic. It was July 21 when we were given the second and final neurologist's opinion. Her method of telling us, of being the voice of confirmation after Dr. K's preliminary diagnosis and requisite first neurologist testing, was to say something like, "You know what others have told you... well..." with her words sliding into a silence that was supposed to let us know the worst. Most likely this woman was a high-achiever through all of her education. Certainly, like a badge of honour, she wore those terrible shoes that female medical specialists almost always wear: cheap black pumps. I remember being distracted by them, wondering why, when one has a decent salary, they can't buy something beautiful to make their day more pleasurable. A little leather something from Spain or Germany or France really does make a day, in my experience. There's just a cruelty to ugly and cheap pumps. Hers made her look like Minnie Mouse... was the adolescent thought in my head. Do women who wear them think they're sexy? I was dying to ask. But instead I asked her how it was she knew Marty's ALS wasn't CIDP—something I'd read about—or some other neurological condition. Her relief at my questioning was so obvious, it was painful. It put her back into her own water, and she swam in gleeful circles, explaining how the diagnosis worked, how she would determine it was not other possibilities. I half-listened, and wondered at myself trying to create a comfortable place for this woman who should take it upon herself to go to a drama class and learn how to tell people shit news. Don't they have drama classes in the science and medicine faculties? Through it all, my heart was breaking. I was absorbing that, on some level, I—we—had been hoping, hoping, hoping. Now our first task, or mine, would be to share this with our boys, and I'd have to do better than Minnie Mouse.

Then, on yet another level, I knew that deep inside myself was some strange recognition that this was life, this was how it was to be. It didn't mean not to fight it, it didn't mean to accept, but it did, and it did. Not for the first time, or the last, did I have that sense of holding on to disparate thoughts, thoughts pulling in opposing directions, and the need to do just that: hold on. One can need to be, and feel, many things at one time, all the time. I was learning that that is what, in part, causes the exhaustion of caregiving.

The neurologist left the room at one point, which was a relief. Marty and I could hold each other and talk. Except at that moment there seemed nothing to say. It was a moment we'd both been awaiting. And expecting. He stayed on the chair where he was sitting when she'd delivered the news, and I leaned over and wrapped my arms around him from behind. I could feel him shaking. Words didn't seem capable of carrying anything right then.

It wasn't until an evening, several days later, with a couple of visiting friends on the back deck, that the word came up. Over barbecued burgers, and the friends' plans to host a fundraiser, suddenly the words were there. "I'm dying," said Marty. "Oh, don't say that," said our friend quickly. Her eyes filled with tears—a first, in my memory. But moments later she said something rippingly funny, as was her wont. And there was relief in that. It wasn't a time to discuss. Maybe, for him, it was a moment of trying on the reality. I had that sense myself, so often. Is this us? Is this real?

After the friends went home, I tried for a thread of conversation that might take the two of us back to that word. How to bring up the subject? We started to talk about one of our sons, and soon Marty was in tears. The emotional quality of ALS, the tears that had become always close to the surface, made it hard to talk. I let the moment go. I had to. There was such potential for cruelty, it seemed. I felt as I did when his father spent a week in the hospital years before, after a series of heart attacks, then passed away, and through it all Marty shared almost nothing of his emotions with me. I felt on the outside, not allowed in.

THE CLINIC FOLKS gave us time to absorb the news and work with our family doctor, and in mid-August we returned for our first "Team Visit." By then I'd read the Oxford handbook twice and gained knowledge that would be useful throughout the months ahead. Much of it terrified me, but I felt better for the knowing.

ALS has something like cruise control—it sets it, and moves by it. If it starts out at 50 kilometres per hour, it progresses the same. Likewise, if it takes off at 180 kilometres per hour. Marty's ALS must have been set at 250.

No one at our clinic ever shared such information. Perhaps they saw no value in it. I was, after all, an old history major, and something of a self-diagnosed research bitch. I took solace in books and bites. Many didn't, I suspected, and I understood why.

For the first team visit, they came in two-by-two, first the dietician and the speech specialists, both kindly but mildly patronizing. Both leapt onto favourite hobby horses: one about eating foods that won't cause choking (we weren't there yet, and didn't want to think about it), and the other, once Marty admitted struggling with speech and volume, insisting on the wonders of an amplifier. She brought it up several times during the appointment, and this was one of the first times of many like this. I came to recognize this theme of people—both in health care and in other spheres—making suggestions. In general, it wasn't the suggestions themselves that were irritating, but the insistence, evidenced by the repeating of the idea, and the tone of having discovered the source of something akin to cure, when in fact the suggestions were not helpful, or seemed not to be based in our immediate reality. Later, I became better at recognizing genuinely helpful ideas, or at least the people whose thoughts were based in logic and in our needs. I also became better at recognizing the others, those with outlandish ideas, and I would head them off to the side, and leave them there sputtering. But I tried to keep open; after all, I didn't know what was in Marty's mind. It was never me dying, and I had to respect that. I was the side-man.

One specialist was using a Blackberry, I remember—an antique to Marty's mind. He'd always loved the technological latest. He commented, she responded, and I in turn joked. I was so used to how his mind worked. It meant there was still this connection between us. It meant we were both still alive. But the clinicians looked taken aback by my joking. I remember wondering at this, thinking they'd be hungry for any levity in their day. Or did they have moments when they had to check their own, maybe thinking that humour from their end would not be appropriate or appreciated?

The next two were the physiotherapist and the occupational therapist who'd been so kind about emailing me photos of renovated bathrooms. It was good to meet her face-to-face. The physiotherapist tested Marty's hand strength, and spoke and recorded numbers without any explanation of what the numbers meant. My Internal Research Bitch wriggled in consternation, and I had to remind her to chill. Before they left, we were asked if we were still sleeping together. Marty could still walk and talk, I wanted to point out. And sex organs are on the list of what doesn't "go." I resisted the urge to say something else funny. But they made me sad, with their earnestness. And the lack of any follow-up to the question. Why ask?

I went out to add time to the parking meter and returned in the middle of a full-blown discussion on antidepressants. Marty talked about it on the way home, and it felt to be a life preserver thrown into our waves. Or his waves, anyway. I was bumping up alongside the boat while clutching the life preserver, with no ladder or rope in sight to actually get out. Again, my internal dialogue (she is so loud!) questioned: What could it hurt? Not for the first time, I recognized the sadness that was growing in my spouse. Marty never had been particularly introspective, and he didn't speak directly to what he was feeling now. His enthusiasm for the topic of medication was a revelation.

But before the drive home, and after the OT/ physio team, came the social worker. This was the only team member on his own. Was the choice of a male deliberate? I listened to him talk about personal resources, accessing how one has dealt with "bad times" in the past, how that knowledge can be used again, how one should "live for the day." Did he really believe that this applied to the reality of dying? Had anyone ever pointed out to him that we have one mouth and two ears for a reason? Listen. *Please listen.* When he discovered Marty was a musician, he told us about the type of music he himself listened to—radio pop—and didn't ask what Marty played or taught. He didn't ask other questions that might give him some knowledge of this person sitting in front of him. He didn't ask what was important to Marty, what made him feel good, what he first thought when he woke up, did he dream at night, heck, did he sleep well? Anything that might lead to a useful place, instead of telling him to "live for the day." I imagined it as a hand-crafted wooden sign in a cabin loo, something with a roll of Star Wars toilet paper beside it. Kitsch.

At first, when the social worker began to speak, I felt some relief. I'd been struggling to find opportunities to push conversation beyond talking about the daily practicalities.

Maybe we could crack below the surface and the conversation might carry on at home. Marty might share what was in his mind. But this didn't happen.

He looked at the clock through the social worker's words, and said something about golf. I finally stopped the fellow and said my husband had a tee time, and we needed to go.

"But you have others to see."

No. There was a tee time.

This happened at the next appointment too, in September, on a gorgeous sunny day. Again we were told there were others to see. The appointment at that point had already been more than two hours. They were unhappy about the tee time. In the summary they sent our doctor, it was noted that the "client... wishes to leave his clinic appointment for a scheduled golf game." There was something of a put-out tone to the words.

Death over sunshine! Hard to imagine why anyone would want to cut short this time of discussing pending death, with a mere golf time waiting. Hard to choose, and to choose correctly.

That September tee time was one of Marty's last times on the course.

For days after these clinic appointments, I questioned myself, second-guessing how judgmental I'd been of the specialists' ways. I came to dread the visits. The hour drive each way, the hours of questions and answers that, for the most part, I already knew from my research. Those days each took away or diminished maybe as much as a week of Life. ALS never moves backwards. If you allow yourself—the patient—to experience exhaustion, there is no "resting up" that will restore you. For all intents and purposes, that time is lost. ALS is unlike MS, with its fluctuations, forwards and back, when a person living with it can be using a walker for some weeks then return to using a single cane; and it is also unlike Parkinson's which must be worked at with exercise and daily effort (Parkinson's, ALS, and Alzheimer's are related neurological conditions).

Our last visit to the Clinic was supposed to be in the second half of January. By then, it was such effort getting in and out of the car that I emailed to ask if there was any way we could do the visit remotely, via Skype possibly, and was told no. However, I knew that what we were offered by the Team in all our earlier visits could, for the most part—and especially in latter stages—be replicated remotely.

In those late summer days and early fall, we took Marty's questions about antidepressants to Dr. K, and he said Marty could try them, but that the part of the brain affected in ALS is often just not a good fit with these medications. The ALS brain does not accommodate many meds, truly, even sleeping meds. Maybe he realized the placebo effect might be useful, though, and didn't say no. When Marty did take some a short time later, he found it even more depressing that there wasn't a noticeable change in his spirit.

Clinic visits were a chore. But some part of me recognized the strange silver lining of a terminal disease that comes with little one can do. This wasn't borne of laziness, but of my resistance to the constant poking and prodding of contemporary life. We do have a collective urge to over-examine so much that won't matter, in the end. Maybe it's so much distraction, from the creating of a well-lived and genuinely examined life.

22

Distraction

BEFORE THAT PERIOD of a last falling-in-love, there were many years between us that weren't between us, a time when we lived separate lives. Occasionally, in the midst of changing a diaper or assisting with homework or finding myself watching Martha Stewart at 10:35 PM once again—alone—it would occur to me that maybe my marriage needed some work. Then I would focus on ensuring there was nothing left in a fold in a toddler's groin, or on the explanation of long division to a grade-school son, or on the fact that Martha appeared to have plunked on more poundage. Life would sail on.

Distraction.

Meanwhile, my husband distracted himself with more golf, followed by longer nineteenth holes, and more friends.

In those last couple of years, when we did stumble into each other again, when we found we were still there, it was a surprise to me to realize that he enjoyed coming home from the golf course to the deck, to sit by the fire, with a ready glass of wine. It seemed that once the distraction was over, gone, and we could surrender willingly into something else, there was something else to explore. That surrender seemed significant to me. The willingness more so. The exploration, perhaps most. I wondered, at moments, and hardly began to articulate even to myself, what it might mean to surrender and explore where we were now. Not necessarily to accept, but not to fight against the grain of our lives either; to embrace that this was it, this was our life and lives. When I stopped pushing against the grain, against what was happening, there was some undercurrent that this was, somehow, as it was. "Supposed to be" was a phrase I didn't want to approach, but it was there nonetheless.

Once this corner was taken, though, the corner of being ill and diagnosed, Marty put distraction into place again: the television was turned on, rarely off. Sometimes the television sound was simultaneous with the radio. Night-time reading was eschewed for podcasts, though Marty realized that for some months leading to diagnosis, reading had been a struggle of comprehension. But his ears were never not filled with sound. Once he could no longer teach guitar, mid-August, he was never far from his computer, with Facebook and emails, and he always, always had phone in hand. He never ignored a beep or ding.

Having experienced what it was, once, to turn down distraction and enter into something—our relationship—might it occur to him to enter into his new reality?

The idea of "enter into" seemed different from surrender. Surrender had connotations of acceptance, a degree of giving up. In our society, hockey fights cancer and daffodils fight cancer. Ice water and buckets fight ALS. Not to fight is not acceptable.

So there seemed to be a cruelty to my thoughts on this. Who was I to suggest we enter into? After all, did I want to enter into—immerse myself in—the role of caregiver? Oh, I balked at that thought. The balking itself gave me perspective.

I tried to open a conversation about this, and Marty interrupted by telling me about how a particular golf-mate came up with the best distracting questions. I asked how that worked, and he shared some of the questions of that day. As he was speaking, I realized he was challenging me to do the same.

For weeks, almost from that first day, I'd been aching for and seeking out an opportunity to talk about what all of this meant. Even in part. But it seemed impossible to broach the subject. I could bring up topics of everyday care and practicalities, but beyond that, to try to speak of what surrounded us, and what it meant to be dying, he would let me know not to go there by quickly veering off to another subject, or checking his phone, or even physically moving away, leaving the room to go to his studio. Too often he'd turn on the television, and invite me to spend another evening on the couch watching some series. Sometimes I just wanted to turn it off and say, "Let's talk."

Instead, I found myself letting it be, thinking that if it were important to him, and he was comfortable with it, words would come. Two people, two sets of needs.

Months later, when so many muscles had shut down, he developed a way of closing his eyes with a slow sweep and looking away dismissively. The message was clear. *I don't want to talk about it.*

This element of caregiving—tough conversations—made me ponder the complexity of being care-recipient. *Tougher to receive than to give,* came to mind.

In not talking about our reality—shared and otherwise—there seemed to be a danger. How were we going to get through this if we didn't open it up and look at it? Yet why would we? We'd never talked enough about things that were under the surface. I hadn't realized until then how little time we'd spent in this way. We took full advantage—too much so—of the ease that can come with an established relationship. "We've said everything we need to," Marty had said more than once in the past. But had we created a culture of silence between us?

Can two people know each other that well? Easy comfort takes away from the dynamic possibilities in an old connection. Old connections sometimes need to be fired up, blown up even. But this was beyond blowing up.

It began to seem to me that, as much as the caregiver had tasks, the caregiven had work, too. I wasn't sure exactly what that might be, though. It would look different for everyone. What might it mean for me someday?

There are types of work that are significant to who we are, work that simply must be done. Becoming human is a wonder-filled burden we carry. Moving from one age to another. Moving to the end.

To leave loved ones knowing they are loved, have been loved, with as clean as possible a pain, might be a significant piece to this human work. Having time with the knowledge that one is leaving this place is some compensation for having to live with that knowledge. Perhaps time can be a gift.

Another significant piece of work is to know one's own soul. I suppose this would be that "Be at peace" or "acceptance," that people speak of. How important is it? What of

Dylan Thomas's *Rage, rage against the dying of the light*? It has its place, too.

This is so individual. Loved ones, knowing the dying one is a rage-person, might appreciate the rage, the resistance to going; it might cause them to feel more loved. The beloved cared enough to fight. Rage might be as soul-building as peace and acceptance. The work would be to know one's self enough to know how to build the soul. Whether by rage or peace, or mix, or... It does seem to me though that, regardless of beliefs of after-life or *whoosh, away in the wind with you*, there is a need to have—and to hold on to—one's soul as one slips out of this place to wherever one is going.

We did once go to a counsellor in those early weeks. But together with the easy tears of ALS, the process of opening up was painful, and Marty walked away from the appointment saying, "I didn't need that."

After, I couldn't shake the feeling of circling outside and around some metaphorical house, a building full of windows and no doors. There had to be one door, I thought. Who knows, maybe he'd already found his way in and poked around these questions on his own, and didn't need me to be with him. Certainly, while I was looking for the entrance to this house, Marty seemed happy enough to be seeking out a putting green in its yard. He didn't seem to need to go inside. Perhaps he had the right idea. We could sit there, together, and watch the sun go down.

Distraction.

23

Hope and
Acceptance

IT BECAME A constant, the move from hope to acceptance and back. There always felt to be shades of each, and fluctuation between. I tried to pry them apart, to separate and examine, but felt like a child taking something to pieces that would never go back the same. There were days of more one than the other, and then moments that moved so completely, so quickly, that I was lost.

I tried to look acceptance in the face, whatever that might mean. Then stepped back. I tested waters of each with Marty; which was the right temperature today? Like dipping an elbow into the bathwater of a baby. In which, or which combination, could we swim?

One day in August he returned from a golf game, and he was buoyed by hope. The woman he golfed with in partner games had suggested he ignore the diagnosis completely, and he had decided she was quite right. He'd set himself beyond hope to ignore. Also, she shared with him the work of a remarkable naturopath who could heal everything. This man had a practice one tunnel and two bridges away, and was worth every dollar one could spend.

I researched this person to discover he was a bowel specialist, working with people living with Crohn's disease and other digestive and abdominal disorders.

But at the moment of speaking of this woman—let's call her Melanie—and her admonition to ignore, I felt a jag of jealousy, not something I was used to.

My feelings were mixed. Part of me wondered at how he could accept far-fetched thinking from another, when I had the feeling that, if I were to articulate any hidden hope on my part, he'd pronounce it as foolish, or reject it in some way. There was some primal jealousy here in me—unpleasant to look at, especially at this point in our lives, and something I'd tried to avoid in our relationship. Why did such have to come out *now*? Heightened emotions? Everything feeling sharpened and waiting, with some ugliness in the "sharpened"? Followed quickly by frustration. I'd tried to talk with him about what was happening, and how we might live with it. Maybe not "ignore," but something of "push back." I'd always disliked the "fight disease" thing. There was something about the idea of fighting one's own body that had never sat right with me. But a push.

Aren't our bodies intrinsic? Psychological, emotional, mental healing—to my mind—was so connected to our body, that I believed one could work almost entirely on the body, and the emotional would follow. I'd done this in my own life. Just hauled my bum to yoga class for months, not analyzing the process, letting it happen... and it did.

In the first days after diagnosis, all I wanted to do was gather Marty's body in my arms, and cry for it and comfort. I wasn't angry with his body; I had no desire to fight.

But here someone else had handed him the idea of ignore, and I, as spouse, had to scrutinize my own feelings about this. How could such a thing bother me? If this was useful to him, I should be glad. Maybe what was really bothering me was the enthusiasm with which he embraced the idea. My weeks-turning-into-months of ideas or plans felt more of the "doctor prescribing" sort. Somehow—how and when?—I'd become a spectacularly pragmatic person. A person of do and not dream. Batwoman. I thought to shake her off. Even as I wondered at how to use this mental space of ignore.

Within hours of talking about it, I did have to admit that the cloud under which we'd been living had indeed lifted. While it may still hang somewhere over us, it was high enough overhead not to be seen, not to cast quite the shadow it had.

We had close to a week like that, under the spell of ignore. Yes, it was bliss. Or as blissful as could be. We used that time to revert to the types of conversations that ignored the basket of supplements in the middle of the table. And to laugh easily. It became a secret to hug to ourselves. We were able to sit through a visit with Dr. K, in which I found myself thinking, "You don't know… this isn't happening! We are all right!" (Yes, it's true. How does this happen? Because we want it to.)

The days slipped by, and ignore shifted to hope again (was signing the local non-miraculous naturopath's paperwork part of that?), until there was an evening by the fire, when Marty broke down, and tearily admitted he would do anything not to be facing the outcome. He said that already his golf game was going, and he was feeling so physically weak. So ignore did only happen because we wanted it to.

My heart had to break its not-even-dried glue all over again. (Who am I kidding? There was no glue. It was just spit.) I realized how I too had wanted the pretence. Could there be somewhere in between?

I finally talked about the research I'd been doing. I actually felt some gratitude toward Melanie because, on some level, her advice was what had brought this to a head, brought him to a place of saying he'd try. He hadn't actually said that before this point. There was a guy in Australia who'd lived with ALS for ten years, I told Marty. Finally able to share. This is what this Aussie guy's been up to. I didn't share that this fellow readily admitted the diagnosis might be a bit off. I also shared thoughts on liver health; maybe his drinking could be cut back—at least, for the sake of a clearer mind. Alcohol, even just a beer or two, had been affecting him for almost a year now; we could see that retroactively. He nodded, and talked about stopping vaping, which maybe wasn't as innocuous as proponents would have us believe. Maybe not, I said, tentatively, scarcely able to believe we were having this conversation. Three times he said, avowedly, that he'd do anything.

Cleve loomed in the doorway, and Marty asked him to fetch another beer.

So maybe the plan would start tomorrow.

I was torn. When struggling for life, do you focus on health—meaning, do you listen to every piece of advice or information, and strive to act on it? Or do you simply—if I can say simply—enjoy life, what there is of it, and every last moment? And how might you interpret this? What does it mean, even, to use words like "struggle" and "enjoy?"

Marty wrapped up the evening by planning for a new diet, new, new, new. "I'll do anything," he repeated. I found myself excited. Full of hope. Forget acceptance.

Even before he was up the following morning, I was at the store, buying The List—purified water, grapeseed extract, and the highest quality green tea—the only thing I ever found documented in research, with its component of EGCG.

We ate breakfast. He was heading out, once again, to golf. We had plans later for a nine-hole game with two other couples. I would join him, was the plan.

I suggested that maybe, instead of seeing this quitting as forever, it might be best to think of it as for a month. I said this because, after twenty-seven years, I had some idea of how he dealt with such things. But even so I wasn't prepared when he looked at me in surprise and said, "I can't quit anything *today*! Today is party day!"

Something in me went sink-and-thud when I heard this. What was that "I'll do anything" about?

No, what I was feeling was more than *sink and thud*; it was sheer anger. It rushed into me from some place I'd rather not think about, a wave of utter exhaustion. I realized not much was keeping me upright. Moments after Marty had been picked up to go to the course, I was in my car, running errands, and as I drove the highway, I found myself screaming at the top of my lungs. It wasn't the first or last time the car was a refuge for such. Ah, the fricative of a certain word that just feels good coming out. How was it that I had spent hours, days, weeks inside books, online, phoning, asking, asking, asking, trying to find ways to live with this? How was it to feel things become dust in my fingers, and watch as the wind swept them away? To hear laughter—at me and hope. Fuck hope. I even thought, *Fuck you.*

Then went home and made quinoa salad of my guilt. Ignore was never a real option.

Later, when I joined him on the golf course, I was brought up short by the realities of his new game. He stumbled and tottered. His putting was the one and only element that could at all be relied upon. On hole number five, I made a quick trip to the little toilet shed, wiped my eyes and blew my nose, humbled and quieted by the courage he showed on the greens, just trying to enjoy his game. His party day.

I DID PERSIST after that, with some quiet research. I researched clinical studies, but discovered that one needed to have been diagnosed at least a couple years before taking part. So I focused on what was at hand, and through the summer, I acquired reasons for daily Epsom salt foot baths. Cilantro made it to the table most days. With avocado and sardines at times. The basket of supplements was filled, emptied, and filled again. So much ritual. Did any of it matter? Perhaps not, but if I missed a piece, if I so much as forgot a Vitamin D drop, Marty called me on it. Was this acceptance or hope? By end of summer, I was adding nasty-tasting chlorella/spirulina green stuff to the potion, and experimenting with apple juice as pectin is, apparently, supposed to have amazing properties. One day in late August, he swallowed the juice, looked at the pieces of apple, and asked, "Is this going to make me better?" We both began to cry, and I went to the bathroom, where I honked and wiped before coming out. I said, "It's what I'm good at." I didn't add that it is what I'd discovered I'm good at. I had so wanted to be good at other things. Minutes passed. Then I asked him if he wanted me to stop doing this as I was. No, he said. I said that I was hoping maybe it would slow the process, or at the very least, give him a clearer mind—his mind was so foggy, and had been for months, we'd realized. He nodded.

I asked, too, if my organizing of the house, my research, my attention to food, my sense of *task*... did it all come across as not caring? I wasn't falling apart emotionally. At least not on the surface. Care and lack of care could take surprising forms; I was so aware of that. Again, he said, "No."

Did he understand that it was my way to hold on? He seemed to.

Maybe mostly it was me who wondered.

24

Mary &
Martha

THE SENSE I had at the outset, that we were still us, was beginning to feel over-populated. There were perhaps too many of me.

There was this irritating me—the one who organized and understood the need to think about tomorrow and plan for next week, and even take a peek at what might be required of me a month from now. The one who even knew to turn off my brain (or tried to) if thoughts went beyond next week or month. She was necessary. But she made me squirm. Because I wanted to be someone else—a loving spouse, or artist daydreamer. Or at least someone who could dream at night, asleep. This other person I was revealing myself to be seemed incapable of anything beyond list-making and research and careful cooking.

To my mind came the Biblical story of two sisters, Mary and Martha, and their brother, Lazarus.

I grew up with those stories. Every Sunday my father opened that big book with its magic of old English and read. The stories embedded at cellular level. It's the figure of Mary, at Jesus's feet, listening to his words, that was imprinted on my mind, as it is in many minds of those growing up in Christian faith. I don't know how that image resonates with boys and men, but as a girl it spoke to a hierarchy of tasks.

It is surprising to return to the actual text and discover the words from which church leaders have extracted these guiding thoughts, and images. The sisters are evoked in such brief verses, a handful of words, that have been expounded upon, dissected, painted by artists, interpreted, and re-envisioned. There are several vignettes in the books of Luke and John that show us the sisters, Martha intent on making and serving food, and Mary sitting at Jesus's feet, listening, rapt.

The verses in the book of Luke say that Martha was "cumbered about much serving," and approached Jesus, and said, "Lord, dost thou not care that my sister hath left me to serve alone? bid her therefore that she help me." And Jesus answered: "Martha, Martha, thou art careful and troubled about many things: But one thing is needful: and Mary hath chosen that good part, which shall not be taken away from her."

In another story, Mary "took a pound of very costly oil of spikenard, anointed the feet of Jesus, and wiped His feet with her hair. And the house was filled with the fragrance of the oil." She even took some grief from a disciple who thought she shouldn't have spent the money on the ointment.

I wanted my house to be filled with that fragrance. After all, given the choice between a foot massage and kitchen work, I'd take the massage. And Jesus said that Mary's listening was "that good part" of the sisters' actions. In churches, even in the family Sundays of my growing up, that message of taking time to listen to Jesus, to make him the centre, was held up as the model. Martha was the woman in the kitchen, away from the saving words and mired in chores and daily grind.

I have long held images and notions in my mind about these two and, as others have, I've tried to grapple with their significance and meaning. Was it possible there was some sustenance left in these ancient stories? I'd long ago put aside the bindle-stick of paradigms that seemed to belong to my childhood.

As a caregiver, these two women began to visit my mind, heart, and soul regularly, sometimes separately, sometimes together. In my heavier months of caregiving, they just showed up without being asked, and stepped through the doorway—Martha with a look of superiority in her unflagging energy, and Mary with such accusation: What was *wrong* with me that I didn't understand that love—simple love—had all one needed to get through? All you need is love.

You don't understand, I wanted to say. To both.

What about a third sister, one with shared qualities and more? But no. The stories, at first, seem to have a reductive nature; humans tend to like either/or. For our children, we call it choice therapy. It's supposed to ease life.

I have looked at areas of my life in my past, and wondered whether I am one or the other. As a wife, I've ached to be Mary. But more often, as a mother of three, working in and out of home, I've had to be Martha. You know Martha wives and mothers. We're the ones who opt to be designated driver with one glass o' red, no more, over taking a cab and figuring out a way to retrieve the vehicle the following day. We make meals that result in real leftovers for next-nights when there are multiple sports or music lessons. And we know how to make leftovers tasty, and how to keep straight in our minds and on our calendars all those classes and practices and games, alongside our own work schedule.

Martha is capable and convenient. But even as a writer, Mary has been my go-to desirable—the bohemian, the artist, the one who eschews the everyday concerns and can spend hours looking out the window. Mary indulges. And I am pulled towards her. Then, too, that commendation of Jesus. No small thing. I've heard about it often, sitting in a pew. Mary hath chosen that good part.

Though, left entirely to Mary, would the words get on the page?

I let that thought drift away.

In the third story, Martha goes out into the town to find Jesus because their brother, Lazarus, has died, and she wants to ask Jesus why he did not come earlier when he might have saved him. Mary stays home to grieve. In this story, Martha affirms her faith. Jesus reassures her. And he resurrects Lazarus from the dead. This story is less often told from the pulpit.

In the days following Marty's diagnosis, I found that point of acknowledging that this was an opportunity to show him what he meant to me. It was, to my mind, the highest calling of love: to care until the end. In Leonard Cohen's words, *Dance me through the panic 'til I'm gathered safely in / Lift me like an olive branch and be my homeward dove / Dance me to the end of love.*

In my journal, through the months, are notes of almost prayer: *Let me feel our connection through this. Let me be there when he goes. Give me the good to remember, and to sustain through the inevitable pain.* Yes, the panic.

No one said to me, "You are a romantic idiot!" If they had, I would not have listened. Who would be brave enough to say that to someone trying to face a recent terminal diagnosis? Would I? Even now? People do say, all the time, "This *will* draw you closer together than you've ever been," which is, to my mind, a spectacularly stupid thing to say—to assume. But at the outset it seemed possible, desirable.

These people generally added words about this idea being based on observation of their grandparents' marriage, forgetting that they were nine and a half at the time, and there is so much that children miss—willfully so, perhaps—about adult connections and misconnections.

So caregiving might begin with Mary, but what about Martha, with her wide hands and square-tipped fingers, broad in hip and shoulder? Her lips are full; she prefers to smile than not, and her smile is open and free of guile. She's lost the art of flirting and seduction. Long ago she depended on being young for that, but now she counts on someone liking her hand-tossed pizza. I wouldn't be taken in by her pizza.

Mary, Mary, Mary, with your slim hips. Let me follow you. Show yourself.

Even as both called to me, I knew in my gut that it was Mary I wanted to follow, if I had to choose. If I could choose.

25.

Team 3

WE SOLD OUR car with standard shift. I mentioned that it would make sense for us to buy Cleve's car; he'd bought another, a vintage Lexus he'd purchased to share with his dad, while Marty could still drive, he said, after a lifetime of practical beater cars. But Cleve had taken good care of his Camry, and it would make sense to buy this Toyota, and get rid of the old standard shift that was rapidly becoming a challenge for Marty to drive. We didn't speak directly as to why we would get rid of it.

Marty listed our car online, and received calls throughout that afternoon, and then in the evening, when we were sitting around the fire, someone came with a strong flashlight to look under the hood in the late-day shadows, papers and cash ready in hand, and drove it away.

I heard it rattle off down the road, and then Marty appeared around the corner, hundred-dollar bills in hand, happy for the sale. My heart was in my gut. But we sat down by the fire, poured more wine, listened to more music.

I went with Cleve to do the changeover paperwork to purchase his car. It was easier if I did it, in my name. We never talked about that. I just did it.

As the next few weeks passed, several times I heard myself referring to the Camry as "my car." Each time I did, it brought me up short. What was happening to the word "our"? This word "my" felt strange. Yet it slipped out so easily. The strange was instantaneously there, in the air, but after the fact. *My.* How could something be my? It was as if some other part of me had gone off to the store, and in a tight corner change-room, was trying on something. Did it fit? Did I have to wriggle into it? Did it look horrible? Would anyone recognize me? Worse, would I recognize me? What if I didn't want to try it on? Yet had to buy it. I could just take it home, wait until I absolutely *had to* wear the thing, then pull it on, without passing a mirror, and walk out. I worked hard to remember to say, "our car." It was still our car, even if he drove it less and less. It was our car to drive him around. The trunk of our car fit the wheelchair quite nicely we discovered as I—we—drove the six hours to Portland to celebrate our last anniversary together.

Our car. Was a very very very fine car.

26

Mr. Fireman

THERE WAS AN evening midsummer. Marty and I had a salmon dinner outside with the chiminea going, crackling on its hearth. There had been some real rain the day before—the only all summer so far, such a dry year—and I'd run a hose under the deck for more moisture, and it felt safe. Really, the municipality had long ago created a bylaw about open fire, but there seemed to be an understanding if people were reasonable about it and took precautions. Throughout the summer, I was mindful of Marty's wish for this summer to be normal: golf, Rock School, evening fires.

Emmett was home. He joined us, spoke of Steely Dan and lyrics. Ole arrived home from being out on the river with his buddies. Later it was growing dark, and Cleve returned home to share his workday.

I settled into the evening, surrounded by my family, and so aware of that. With Cleve moving out soon, such evenings were finite in number. We were rich for this one. I'll admit to some residual bit of hero in me. Batwoman. Rescuing an hour. The hammock was swinging with Emmett. Faces were illuminated by flames. Music, wine, talk, laughter.

Then I realized there were also sirens and flashing lights. The street out front was filled with noise. The noise had come to a stop. Right outside our house.

It took me a half-second to realize what this meant, and I dashed into the house, filled a large jug of water, poured it over the fire, and repeated three more times, until all that was left was hissing steam and grey ash—just as the back gate bumped open, and we were invaded by a burly, ageing fireman flanked by several young worked-out up-and-coming uniformed fellows. The leader marched up the few stairs to the deck and launched into how stupid we were to have a fire on the bare wood of our deck (I numbly pointed out the solid tile hearth underneath), then berated us with, "I'm *sure* you go to sleep while this burns out!" (We don't, I started to say. We sit with it until there is nothing left), and how we needed to know that all around us the province was burning up (and you so wish you were there, anywhere but here, I wanted to say, but this time, kept shut).

He sent one of the young men away to find the hose, and I followed the young man. I was shaking. I tried to say something. What was I hoping to say? *Please let us have our evening. It's another Last Thing, and we need it for memories.*

I said something, I can't remember what, and the young man just said, "Talk to the chief—it's all up to him." I could see him watching surreptitiously as Burly Chief threw around his substantial weight to make his point.

Chief took the hose from the young man and rammed it down the chimney. There wasn't so much as a spark left, but he bellowed for the young man to turn on the water, and then he let it flow and overflow, soggy ashes pouring out onto the deck, as he stood shouting out to us that we were lucky, he wouldn't fine us this time. But next time... there'd better not be a next time, he let us know. All the young uniformed men looked embarrassed now

Every muscle in me felt exhausted watching them troop back down the steps, through the gate, with Chief waving the hose around, his men trailing behind

We stood looking after them, the deck suddenly darkened without the flickering fire, all of us feeling soggy. I had a sudden burst of angry energy swell up and out of me, and shouted, "I guess *someone* hasn't gotten any lately!" But they either did not hear, or knew better than to come back.

Ole looked at me in horror. Surely his mother hadn't said that... had she?

But the following day, telling the story to his friends, that was the first bit that came out. *You won't believe what my mom said.*

Some colour from all the ash grey.

27.

Flying Away

CLEVE HAD BOUGHT his condo in Vancouver in April. The possession date was late June. Then the former owners requested to rent it back for some weeks as they weren't having luck finding a new home. That worked well for Cleve, thinking it'd be best to stay at home a while longer now. Although he worked the long hours of the film industry, arrived home late, left early, it was good to have him for those extra weeks. It delayed another goodbye.

His August possession day came and went. He stayed on with us, deciding to take his time preparing the new place, and further delaying leaving his dad. The seven hundred square feet of new home was painted no less than five different brilliant colours—hot pink bathroom, avocado dining, orange kitchen, lemon living room, red bedroom. Not a place for a hangover. It could take a while to make livable. But at one point he needed some help to pull together the last of the preparations.

Marty was still busy through daytime hours with Rock School. He'd booked the more-experienced students for the last weeks of the summer, so that the actual teaching—demonstrating—would be minimal or none. In spite of his hands not working as they should, he was enjoying it for the most part.

Cleve had to work. So I packed the car with paint supplies and, along with Ole, Emmett, and Cleve's girlfriend, Olivia, spent the day cleaning and painting the condo. Of all the days through all those months, that day stood out: a day we accomplished something visible. It was a Martha task, most definitely, in spite of my attempts not to embrace the ways of that sister.

We returned to our little suburb through rush hour, sweaty, smelly, speckled with rollered paint bliss.

Moving day came, a few days later, possibly the most uneventful first-child-leaving-home ever. We did have a barbecue on the deck, followed by a propane fire—the replacement I'd gone out to buy the day after the incident, this one advertised as a "ban buster" fire. But both the barbecue and the fire were routine. Then came the not-routine moment of Cleve standing from his seat, saying goodbye, giving hugs. And he was gone.

Marty didn't have the strength to follow him all the way down the driveway. I remember, in some part of my mind, having to choose between leaving Marty alone on the deck to say goodbye to Cleve on the driveway, or staying back of the house on the deck.

I could hear my son driving away in his car. There didn't seem to be time to reflect, let alone cry. Inside me, something tore a bit.

Later, before bed, Marty began to cry. And speak. When he spoke through tears, I could barely understand his words, but eventually they came through: "Sad day."

I pushed back at the sense of being overwhelmed. In my own mind I'd been inviting memories of carrying a baby over the threshold of a basement suite twenty-three years ago. "It is a sad day," I agreed.

28.

Blank

Before each golf game, I administer
a Vitamin B cocktail shot
in Marty's ass
The local naturopath
—who admits she can't cure, makes no claims to fame
says she can only—possibly—provide some alleviation
of symptoms—
has told me it is not the end of the world if
one forgets to tap the air out of a syringe

One morning, too much on my mind, I do
exactly that. A bruise shows up instantly
As does the awareness I've caused
more pain. I feel sick with this

Same morning I burn five dollars' worth of quinoa
because I forget it on the stove
cut up tomatoes, and then toss them—along with their
stems—into the compost
Mindlessness
Or mind-full-ness

29.

That Monday

TO WHAT DEGREE was it normal to consider the future? The "after" of this time? Anticipating loneliness was exhausting. I heard Marty breathing at night and then, when his breath quieted, there'd be a glimpse of silent future.

Or listening to him in the shower as I lay in bed waiting my turn. Someday there will not be turns, I thought.

Rehearsed sorrow. Too much? It would be months before I stumbled over the phrase "anticipatory grief." My belly leapt with gut recognition; I knew immediately what that meant.

IN AUGUST THERE was a day. I ended up thinking of is as That Monday. Such a simple thing: Marty went to put detergent in the dishwasher. The box of soap was too heavy for him. I had to take it from him, half-empty it turned out, and sprinkle some into the dishwasher, as he backed away and disappeared into his studio. The way he closed the door behind him told me not to follow. I closed the dishwasher. The machine started to chug, and I sat on the kitchen floor and cried. Struggled to get up from the floor. The rest of the day was one of deep despair. I retreated to the couch on the deck, heavy with grief. That urge to tear my self out of my skin was strong, and didn't leave me all day. I couldn't leave it. The sensation was tangible, and made me miserable. I wanted to follow him into the studio, I wanted to feel connected. I didn't like how he had closed the door between us. But I also needed the time on my own to absorb without letting it spill over him. I was so grateful he had his Rock School kids to busy him all day.

Later, I spoke to Ole about spending more time with his dad—realizing my son was thinking this might be four to five years, and I knew then, after That Monday, that four to five was just not going to be. I could feel it. The online descriptions of this disease might read "average three to four years," but we appeared to be on another trajectory.

A WEEK LATER, early in the morning, still dark, my alarm went off. It was the day to drive Ole to the airport to return to school. He and I put his bags in the trunk, and had breakfast, made coffee. At quarter to five, I awoke Marty to say it was time to say goodbye. Ole followed me into the bedroom and leaned over to hug and kiss his dad. Marty was trying to say something, but was in tears. Ole understood though. "I love you too, Dad," he said.

How could I not have understood those words? How anxious I was, anticipating *not* understanding. Ole had heard exactly what his dad had said to him. I'd heard mumbled sound. My right ear was partially deaf, but my left had no excuse. Somehow, I had to learn the flow to this, even as I resisted the whole. Could I?

I said goodbye too. I'd be back home soon. We were going to the airport long before rush hour. I snugged the blanket around Marty, still teary, and thought back to just a year earlier, when the three of us—Marty and I with Ole—had all flown together to set him up in his school in Oklahoma.

Now one year later, and so anti-climactic. I saw him off at the local airport—*goodbye*—then sat in the car before turning the key to go. This is how it will be now, I told myself. Just Marty and me and Emmett. In our big house. We'd never planned a third child. He'd turned up in a radiologist's photograph; the radiologist had been setting out to track down the fibroids my doctor thought he'd palpated. Cutest fibroid ever, with four limbs and all the right digits.

Now I knew why.

In July I'd run into my friend Vivienne outside the bakery. She'd been widowed years before, when her children were preschoolers. She'd hugged me and told me that someday I would learn the reason behind all this. Those were not words I was ready to accept, not at all—but from Vivienne I had to.

Still, I could only figure out one why at a time. Of course, there were many reasons our third son was in our lives, but this particular one—I would not yet be alone—was significant. That, at least, made sense, when nothing else did. It meant Vivienne might even be right.

That Monday, though, and its week of loss and missing, was a turning point.

30.

Normal

MORNING HAD BECOME my favourite time of day. It used to be the evening. But now I gravitated to beginnings and openings instead of endings and closings. Sleep—the idea of sleep—disturbed me. Like the old nursery-rhyme-prayer: *If I should die before I wake, I pray the Lord my soul to take.* Absurd. It wouldn't happen like that. At least, I thought not. But sleeping did have a lack of control; when the lights were out, who knew what could happen.

Normal shifted week to week, every week. One week Marty insisted he could drive downtown, and he did, with me holding on to the door pretty much all the way. One week later, for the MRI appointment, he casually asked me to drive. So it went.

In the MND handbook, I came across a passage about how the ability to drive a vehicle could extend past a point that seemed possible. I decided not to share that particular snippet. I hugged the reassuring words to myself as Marty continued to drive around our small town for weeks even after his last drive downtown into the city.

Some weeks later, though, my anxiety had risen, and I emailed Dr. K about the driving. I'd stopped riding in the car when Marty drove. Too many times he flew into the driveway and I had to wonder if he could press the brake hard enough to stop. At our next meeting, Dr. K used a few well-chosen words including "insurance" and something to let Marty know not to expect him to defend him if something happened. Marty said he was fine, he was just driving like an old man. Dr. K stepped up with a sharp, albeit funny, answer. I was grateful. Without Dr. K's words, my words were not heard.

We were at the hospital for that MRI, and I looked out from a window to the parking lot below, and remembered that the last time here, looking out at that same parking lot, I was in labour with our youngest, and I could see Dr. K's vehicle pulling up. Felt like a thousand years ago.

On the way out, we talked about the letter I was working on, to my retired-builder father. I was writing to say that we had so appreciated all the house upkeep and renovations he had done for us in the past, but that now he couldn't do this quite like he used to—my brothers and my nephew would need to be the ones to wield the hammers and saws—and he needed to know that we had come to a time to recognize how much we loved him for who he was, not just for what he could do. As I spoke, I realized I could be saying the same words to my husband; he appeared to be taking them in on a more personal level. He nodded. He looked peaceful. I'd hit a mark, a good mark. A mark I hadn't set out to strike. It might not happen the next time I opened my mouth. How long, how often, could I be what I needed to be?

31

Last—
August 16

You don't always know when something is a "last"—
"last" day "last" night "last" meal "last"
student. Her name is Melissa

Marty comes out of his studio, stands
by the doorway, leans into it suddenly, exhausted
"What is it?" I ask
He cries. It comes out: "I can't teach anymore"
He holds out his hands, fingers curling. It's been a long
time really
since they've heard any direction from his head
I hold him. Emmett joins, wrapping arms around both
of us
all of us altogether

The first visit of the at-home physiotherapist
she looks at the line of guitars on the wall
and she says, "I'm so sorry
you've lost this"

32.

Portland
<hr>

IN THE DAYS leading up to this trip, to celebrate our twenty-seventh anniversary, I suggested to Marty that we cut his hair. We'd been watching *Peaky Blinders*, a television series about mobsters, set in Ireland shortly after the First World War, and he'd commented on the haircuts—extremely short sides, with rascally long top. Such clean lines. Reminded me of when we first met, and I was still a hairdresser.

"I can't wear that cut," he said. "My hair is too thin." That's what a barber had told him some time before. It occurred to me that if we coloured it too, then the line of the long top would show up better.

With this suggestion, I could see his old spark, and it warmed my heart.

I went to buy the colour the next day, in a box with a bright-eyed redhead on it.

I liked to think it wouldn't be our last anniversary, but knew that, at the very least, it would be the last with him able to walk.

WE WENT. MARTY with his flaming red hair. Me with my driver's hat on. I had to be so conscious of my driving. I had to elicit his confidence in how I handled the vehicle, to toughen up, be assertive, aggressive even. In short, I had to drive as he always had, in the hopes he wouldn't feel the loss of driving as much as I imagined he did.

At that point it had been about a month since the evening, post-golf, when he'd slammed open the front door of the house, calling out hoarsely for me to come and get the key out of the ignition. He'd driven, but after parking and turning off the engine, his fingers could not remove the key from the vehicle. The anger and fear in his voice had propelled me out to the driveway to pull the key—so easily—from the car.

BEFORE WE LEFT for Portland, I secretly put the wheelchair in the trunk, thinking we could experiment with it in another place, a place that wasn't home, where no one we knew would bump into us. I was reluctant to tell him I was doing this; I'd just see how the time passed, and how each day shaped, and if there was a need. The keeping secrets gnawed at me, and the damage it was doing to the team I'd thought we were. But in the end, it was only a part of the changes.

Each piece of change seemed so big, but more frightening was how "big" seemed to be growing smaller, as each change thrust upon us became part of the new normal. Somehow the big changes had to seem small enough to be do-able.

I had only been to Portland once before in my life, as a young child, driving through en route to California. I'd forgotten this until I saw the large neon Portland sign, and something twigged. There's something quaint and quirky about that sign. I was suddenly mindful of the memory-building nature of this trip.

I'd booked the hotel weeks before over the phone, and let them know that it was an anniversary vacation, and that Marty had ALS, and I wasn't certain how he'd be walking. When we arrived, I parked as close as I could, but exhaustion hit him when we got to the front desk. The woman at the desk gave us our room pass. I had a self-conscious moment carrying all the luggage, taking a piece from the bellman as he attempted to hand it to Marty. We went up to the floor as directed. The room was at the farthest end of the hallway. It didn't help that once inside the room, we realized it was probably the ugliest in the place, with a view of hotel rooftop, building sides, industrial-looking chimneys, possibly the hotel laundry or kitchen. Hardly anniversary setting. Marty had to take a break, sitting on a nearby stiff chair, absolutely done with the exertion of the walk down the hall. I went back downstairs alone to ask for a more suitable room. They sent us out for a couple of hours, while a room directly across from the elevator could be cleaned, and off we went, in a cab, to seek out one of the brew pubs Portland is known for, Burnside Pub.

The sun was shining, and even with the end of summer chill—and there was—it was warm enough to sit outside at one of the communal picnic tables. We ordered a flight of beer, seasonal testers, and took our time with the menu. Usually when travelling, the walk would have been the time-consuming part of the day, the exploring. Now we had to drive or cab, and then sit. So I consciously checked myself to slow down once at the table, feeling the sun on my shoulders, feeling my husband next to me. Home and responsibility felt blessedly far away. "This is good," I said. "This is good," he confirmed.

Menu: sausages, something European and tasty-sounding. And my eyes skimmed for something I would never cook. Bone marrow. "Never had it before." We spoke at the same time.

The waiter almost talked us out of it. He described it as "gelatinous."

"Let's try it anyway," said Marty. "We can share that and the sausages. Why wouldn't you? What other time are you going to try it?"

That made me think. *I need to remember this question.* I put those words into my mind.

The waiter set the dishes in front of us, and Marty smoothly pulled the sausages toward himself, and pushed the marrow in front of me. "That's all for you, honey," he said grandly.

And left me looking at the halves of well-toasted garlic bread and at the... yes, gelatinous... stuff, with crispy seasoned breadcrumbs over it, still in the bone. I'd had no idea it was served this way, but was curious. We had a laugh as I pushed it back into the centre between us, and pulled the sausage alongside. The masses of garlic in the marrow, and the crunch of crumbs made it rather tasty in fact. Though we both agreed we may never order it again. The word "never" felt okay that day; it was a word we would have used before, for exactly the same reason.

I began a conversation with our waiter about Portland and Vancouver, and the three of us talked. The waiter had to ask Marty to repeat some of his words, a few came out fuzzily. Some people might hardly notice. But if you spent time talking with him, you would pick up on something. I was relieved that the waiter didn't question this in any way. He was quite natural with it. Not everyone is, I was coming to know. I know I'm not. If I have to ask someone to repeat too often, I become self-conscious, and begin not to ask.

As I listened to the conversation between the two of them, I recalled how I'd been not so comfortable with Marty's extroverted ways when I first began to spend time with him. He'd always had the ability to make small talk, and to draw out people, and over the years I learned from him. At some point I'd grown from being shy and introverted, and it was in no small part due to my marriage. I hadn't quite put it together like that before.

Someone—another guest at the end of that picnic table—took a photo of us, and in it you can see the mark of ALS on Marty's face, the descent, the slackening of muscles. The "flat face," as Dr. K described it.

We took a cab back to the hotel, ready for our new room, and a nap—necessary, daily—before going out again.

The last night in Portland was spent at the Lucky Labrador. I took a photo of Marty across the table, and with his astonishingly normal smile and eye twinkle, you wouldn't guess that at that moment too many muscles in his limbs were twitching with fasciculations, unstoppable, constant.

We cabbed, we drove. I missed that walking for miles, and Marty's old MO of finding the highest point of a city on day one, and going up for a visual of the city layout. We'd done this in New York and San Francisco. My plan, to do a wheelchair night ride in a strange town, never happened. (Would such a midnight adventure have been Mary? Or Martha? The midnight part, the adventure, could be pure

Mary. The practicality of using the time as a trial run, that would be all Martha.)

I did suggest it. The moment of bringing it up was hard. "Would you want to...?" And his quick "No." I realized he did not want to use that chair until he absolutely had to. I felt a bit sheepish about smuggling it into the trunk and was relieved he had no idea it was there.

We visited most of the brew pubs, and we found a sleep shop, to buy a pillow that would support his shoulders, beginning to ache in the past several weeks. It was easier to do that away from home. We visited a couple of vape shops to find new flavours.

I drove home through rain and heavy Sunday traffic. It took an hour longer than going. Every minute was worth it. Once there, I pulled out the wheelchair when he was not around, put it back into storage, and hid it under the black sheet he'd used as a stage backdrop.

33

Card

Four days before our anniversary is his birthday
In the grocery store I buy
ingredients for
burgers and cheesecake
and look for a card
I read every possibility and realize there is not one
for us
If I go home and come back later—will one read
differently?
But then I'll have to feel this bad all over
again

I am in tears when I pay, and
the clerk
—who knows someone who knows us
in this small town—
gives me a hug

34.

Struggle

I SAW MARTY struggle to pull out a dresser drawer. He said that the weekend in Portland had taken something out of him. Neither of us regretted it. But it had. Reality: it probably cost us a week. ALS only goes forward, and marches on—Pac-Man, eating your days.

Later, I emptied a bookshelf, and took it upstairs and screwed it to the wall, and then went through Marty's clothes. I left those that were conspiring to make dressing difficult in the drawers, and on the open shelves placed only what he needed in piles of two or three—easy to get at. One layer would make it too easy. There was a question of dignity; how to keep it intact as long as possible. Dignity could go to pieces in the details. As do most things in life.

He saw the shelf in the evening when he came to bed. I didn't say anything about it. Much like when I traded our bedside reading lamps, because with just a gentle touch mine went on and off, whereas his required a real twist that was a problem within early weeks. The changes that we had to make didn't bear mentioning after a certain point. Things just needed to show up when they were needed. The time—short-lived—of feeling like a hero had long passed. Batwoman, nascent or otherwise, seemed to have perished. Maybe Martha had mistaken her for a whining mosquito, and caused her swift end with a capable hand.

35.

End of Summer

I WAS OUT getting groceries, stopping in at the liquor store for wine, refilling the propane tank. Chores. At each place I met at least one person I knew, and talked and ended with a hug. With Charlene at the liquor store, in a tight embrace, I realized that I hadn't showered yet. Hadn't had time. Hadn't thought about it. I wanted to go home and stand under hot water.

I could manage one conversation with someone I bumped into out in the world. Yet in our small town, there were so many to bump into. I could almost manage a second conversation, but inevitably, walking away from that second conversation, I'd be shaky, tension growing in my jaw, and a vague fuzzy-headed feeling. Exhaustion, emotion, or both? Time after time, in stores, running errands, I'd see yet a third person approaching. Even a fourth.

I would begin to shake my head as our eyes connected, or even to hold up my hand, a non-verbal "no." I'd explain quickly. Or rather, mumble about being too busy. Or maybe they saw the truth in my eyes—the truth that I just couldn't do it, couldn't have the conversations, rehashing details of our life, and also facing their sadness and bewilderment. Even the fact that so few knew much about the disease, and the blanks in their knowledge needed filling. But not by me.

I hoped they understood. I came to dread the shivery, shaky feeling of meeting people, talking with them, updating them if they felt it necessary, or felt they had a right... their right being their genuine care. I knew that. But it took so long to recover from these meetings. I tried to avert them. At times, I wished I never had to leave my house.

HOW WAS I going to go back to work? I was scheduled to teach two classes for fall term, a small grad workshop writing class, and a large second-year lecture. I dreaded both.

This is how an old person feels, I thought. Not that I could really know. But I did. It would be years—if lucky—before I knew the truth of this. I imagined a point at which I would recognize "I've felt this before." Or maybe "old" really was a state of mind. Why did I think "lucky?"

I had one old great-aunt left, of her family of thirteen, now in her mid-nineties. She missed her siblings, friends, so many she had known. She'd outlived two spouses. Did she consider herself lucky? She was healthy, lived in her own home. She didn't whine about being lonely. She was busy in her garden. She took care of an apple tree that she planted when a beloved grandson was killed in a motorcycle accident. She had a great-nephew and great-grandson who came to her home on weekends, spent the night in the room she painted and decorated for them, and they shared breakfasts together. They shovelled her snow. She continued to be useful. People in her community chatted and deferred to and laughed with her—good to see. I needed to think about this, being old and alone. But we are born alone. What did it mean to be alone? Do we pick up the phone and call someone to join us? Or do we sit with it? Live with it?

The evenings by the fire on the deck grew quieter. Not the comfortable silence of last summer. Just that of not knowing what to say. The imminent return to teaching hung over me. Summer, such as it was, felt like a cocoon. Passing from one moment to the next could cause acute gratefulness for the passed. Was there a chance that the return to work might make me feel some bit of normal, even for a moment here and there?

AROUND THAT TIME, toward the end of summer, I began to feel a turn. No, it was in the early fall. I was not sure of the nature of this shift, or where it was coming from. Perhaps it was just the change of seasons. There's always a sense of loss with that, so it could be quite normal, and nothing to take stock of.

But I was beginning to feel that in addition to losing my spouse, I was losing a sizeable piece of my self, too. I wasn't certain what that meant, at that point in time, or for the future. What piece? Maybe some last vestige of Mary? I could imagine her slim form, slipping through less than a crack in some doorway, out to the street, listening to the sound of a violin or a flute, some music only she could hear, and something she knew she needed to follow no matter what else was going on.

Huzzah huzzah for Mary! She knew how to take care of herself. *Take me with you.*

But she wasn't taking me with her. What would Martha have done? Packed me an August picnic with plenty of protein? Sent me out with a jacket for the looming chill? "Put on an undershirt," maybe she'd have said, like some worrying mother from the times in which I grew up. Lost times.

36.

On the Point

ON A FRIDAY night, a last of summer, the first of September, I drove my youngest son to a campsite at nearby Point Roberts, a little pie-shaped piece of America that dangles from the Canadian border, untouched by the development to the north. (*National Geographic* did a piece on this, described the Canadian side as "strip mall hell," and created a furor in the local paper, and some sad attempts to add sloping rooftops to otherwise flat buildings in an effort to lose the "hell.") Our homeschool group always camped there the first week of back-to-school, and this year I would not be there, but Emmett was, for one night, sleeping in a friend's tent. Strange to drive from the house, ten minutes away, through the border, to the small community, darker without those malls of the Canadian side. I swore the stars were brighter, even though the bright lights of the nearby port still blazed, and the ferry engines going to the Gulf Islands still thrummed.

The campers had the usual fire going—and so many familiar voices. I wished I could set up a tent and stay the night, too. I wished I could indulge in the normalcy of it all.

(There's a phrase: indulge in normalcy.) I was glad Emmett could. He was sixteen. He should have this.

I drove away from the sound of the waves on the beach, the voices of all ages of children playing capture the flag in the blackberry bushes. I smiled at the crazy bravery or stupidity of playing games in twilight blackberry bushes. Oh to be a kid again. Not an adult in the brambles of it all. So important that kids did their kid things, so that when the time came to do adult things, they didn't feel they'd missed something. We need memories to sustain.

When I returned home, Marty was still sitting by our propane fire with his friend, and he had had too much to drink. Part of me felt frustrated with this, and even with his friend for not stepping in. Not a particularly rational thought on my part. But alcohol was hard on his brain. The different feel, from one fireside to this other, nagged at me.

After Marty's friend left, I asked him if this was what he wanted. He gave me a blank look, reminiscent of his mother's rather dementia'd expression at times. Later, when I read of the research that questions the ability of some persons with ALS to read the emotional quality of faces, and hear tones in voices, I thought back to this time. But at that moment, some part of me was adding up how far the disease had progressed, and the few months before Christmas, and family coming... and... and... and. "I think it exacerbates," I said, finally. But he seemed not to care.

I needed a moment to be on my own, so I started upstairs and sat mid-stairs, a moment of complete exhaustion. Of what worth were the effects of alcohol to him? How could we make life worthwhile? Could we? And even, what was I worth to him? Oh, that was a strange thought.

Would I ever experience pleasure again? If I could, would I do so without guilt? The guilt of being the one left behind, alive. Maybe I felt guilt just with that thought.

My son was in a tent with a fire crackling just beyond its flaps, stars overhead, waves lapping. Away from this for the night.

Maybe alcohol was Marty's way of escaping for one night.

When he came to bed after me, I wrapped an arm around him. Life was too short.

37.

A New
Window

ONE NOTABLE THING about our home, with its 1972 "modern" design, was that there were so few windows facing the front and street. There were only a couple of upstairs bedroom windows, and a long narrow one by the front door. Then, as if to make up for it, the back wall of the downstairs great room was glass from floor to ceiling, from one end of the room to the other.

A few years before, we'd cut in another front window, in an upstairs bathroom, and then that summer of 2015, we focused on the destruction and reconstruction of the downstairs bathroom, a powder-room two-piece—cabin-like, with red cedar v-joint, rough tiles around the sink, and an old bureau-mirror on the wall. It had to become a hospital-worthy serious roll-in shower space. And we took the opportunity to cut in a window. This window afforded a view to the world, a view we'd not had before.

One morning, from that window, I saw two small kids heading to school, possibly as young as Grade 1. *Yeah!* for their brave mother, I thought, in our paranoid world. Yeah!

that she let them walk alone, and trust their selves, and trust that the world was a good place to be. Because it was.

I realized it was September. Morning air cooling, no longer summer.

One of the boys had a little Batman backpack that my oldest would have liked.

I watched until they passed out of sight on their sturdy legs.

38.

A Thing

IT WAS A thing from the beginning and even too close to the end: people volunteering information, ideas. Cures, even. Every disease/malady (of any proportion—numb toes even) was analogous to ALS. And it would be shared with me. Even if no one knew exactly what ALS was. I grew used to Stephen Hawking's name being tossed around.

But some suggestions were so in the dark I wasn't certain how people came up with them.

"Chaga tea," said Marty once, looking up from a helpful text.

"Chaga tea?" I said. "Never heard of it."

"Supposed to be good."

"Says...?"

"A friend," he said vaguely.

It was getting difficult to understand him at times, and he kept his verbal output brief, especially towards the end of the day when he tired. So I didn't press further. But at that point I was tiring of the bombardment of helpfuls.

Nonetheless, I dutifully looked up chaga tea, much as a desk-cop might investigate the thousands of leads called in by nosy neighbours.

Chaga tea is used to treat female cancers, specifically breast. Right. Another close fit.

He mentioned it again. This could be a need to feel he had some input. I went and bought it, from the health-food store with the talkative and opinionated owner (who invariably recommended her personal latest-and-greatest for depression no matter what the affliction).

In the store I told the owner that, sadly, I didn't have time to listen to her today, and I paid and left. Her with her mouth hanging open.

Was this a new me?

I added chaga to the morning mix, and reassured Marty he wouldn't have breast cancer, the day's dollop of shadowed humour.

39.

Fall Folding Away—
Scrapbook

#1.

I bought a huge pot of mums to sit by the front door. Dr.
K chatted about them the first time he came and saw. One
day he just showed up, with no phone call beforehand, and
announced he'd be coming over to our house from now on
to save us the weekly trips to his office. I was so grateful
for this.

We talked about the colour of the flowers and the season. I never bought mums, only admired them outside the
grocery store every fall.

When I let my thoughts move forward, to how I would
make ends meet some vague day in the future, I pulled back.
Any number of small things could brighten the day. Today,
it happened to be fall mums, burnt orange.

#2.

The freezer was full—of garden produce, but also with bits
and pieces, large bits and pieces, that others had brought
over. Who gave us a ham? The first of many dishes of

lasagne was in there, homemade and beautiful. Marty's niece from Regina had a funny expression on her face when she heard about it, and then she shared that in their freezer back home they still had lasagne that had been given to them by people when her mother was dying, how they all grew to be so sick of that particular dish.

But at that point, I was glad for anything. Once, toward the end, a lasagne was left on our front step with a card to explain that the donor's mother had also had ALS, and that this was made using her recipe. That was special.

By mid-fall the freezer was a mess, as I'd simply thrown stuff in. It didn't improve. My idea of organizing was to dig around, pull something out, thaw, cook, and eat. It read as an archeological puzzle to times passed. *What were these people doing when?*

Filled with peas and figs and berries and beans from the garden. Every time I opened a package, I thought of summer. It felt to be the last season of... what? What was the word? Words were beginning to escape me unless I had a pen to hold on to.

#3.

Today I found in my mailbox a note from a close friend of many years. In the note she had tucked three twenty-dollar bills for me to buy something for myself. Her kindness made me cry.

Later I received an email from her. An update on her own diagnosis of breast cancer. Her options were lumpectomy and radiation, or no radiation and removal. No mention of reconstruction. Maybe they didn't consider that for fifty-seven-year-old single women.

I suddenly felt as if something was so terribly wrong that I couldn't even think about this, with a close friend. I was so entrenched in my own proximity to illness that I couldn't get a plane ticket and go spend time with her.

#4.

In the town newspaper, there was a piece about a fundraising event at a local business, Billie's Barbershop. But in the article Marty's tricky surname was mis-spelled, and the altered name distanced me, and left me wondering about the headline: "Family with ALS." Who were these people in this article?

#5.

I found myself folding away summer dresses. I've always loved summer dresses, cooling, feminine. I'd been reluctant to put them away, but I hadn't worn them for several weeks. Looking at them was making me as sad as putting them away. Maybe more so. Increments of sad.

I folded them, the ones I'd bought myself, and old favourites that Marty had brought home for me from a summer work-trip some years before.

Next summer, who will I be?

40.

Django Fest, Whidbey Island

WE DROVE—I DROVE—TO Whidbey Island, Washington, to go to Djangofest, an annual celebration of gypsy guitar players. We stayed at a B&B, close to the small townhalls where the festival took place, but not close enough. Just days before, we'd received the handicapped parking permit in the mail. Such an odd thing in my hands. Mom had wondered if they—she and my father— needed one, and here I had one. We could have used it in Portland.

It came in handy. We could slide into those nearest spots wherever we were; it should have felt better than it did.

The night we arrived, we went to a pub for handmade pizza and beer. Reminiscent of the time in Portland. But this time the bartender assumed Marty had already had enough to drink with his increasingly slurred speech and physical awkwardness. I steeled myself: we owed no one an explanation or apology.

The next day we were doing our morning routine. I was helping him dress, which didn't require too much of me at that point. Buttons usually. I was suddenly aware of a momentary sense of "settled." These felt to be brief times of relief from the unrelenting change. Then, in the next moment, when I was helping him button his cuffs, there was a second when we caught each other's eyes, and broke down and held each other.

The moments flowed thus, in exhausting verticals. It reminded me of the febrile convulsion that our eldest son had as a toddler: it wasn't the degree of temperature that caused the convulsion. It was all in how quickly his temperature rose. So we felt to be emotionally spiking throughout the day, mental convulsions.

On Whidbey, for four days and three nights, Marty did afternoon naps. We headed back to the B&B, and I settled him in, and then went to sit outside in the cooling September sun, writing. Or trying to. It was so hard to focus. But equally so for reading. Sometimes, I just set aside the page and pen, and closed my eyes, and let the sun soak into me. Listened to my breathing as I used to in yoga. My body was stiffening with the lack of regular stretching and exercise. I tried to ignore it, but it was. It creaked and groaned at me.

When he awoke, I amused him by mentioning the angry chipmunk just outside: "Sounds like a faulty fan belt!" His chuckle was something I strove for. Humour lifted us out of our day.

The last performer we saw at the festival was Bireli Lagrene, his first time playing in America. We were so fortunate. We'd ordered the tickets back in June. At one point, I happened to look over at Marty's hands, clapping, and it was as if all the sound in the crowded room melted away, and all I could hear was his clap, and there was nothing there. The hands of one musician applauding another. His rounded hands, no strength left in them to create a sound, yet still he put them together to acknowledge the music. I wrestled my tears not to flow and noted the music and the pleasure it brought. Maybe that was the moment that music became my drug of choice for grieving. It has that power.

I found my mind wandering after the concert, as we headed to the B&B. How could almost thirty years with another person feel to be so much less than that? I sifted through memories, and there did not seem to be three decades. Years of being too busy seemed to have vanished, unlived. Time had a quality to it that seemed to stretch and shrink in alarming ways. I considered how often Marty had come to Djangofest without me; this was the first time I had accompanied him. He'd otherwise come alone, and spent time with other players drawn to this gypsy music, or he had come with a guitar-playing friend. So many years we'd had our separate lives. So many years I spent as a full-time working mother with young children. Should I have spent more time with my spouse? Yet, where would my relationships with my boys be if I had? I was going to need those relationships in the not-so-far future. Also, all the time Marty'd spent developing friendships as his extroverted personality required... now that came around in the shape of so many friends willing to raise funds to assist us through this. If I was the one who was ill, what would that look like? Strange question, I thought. Possibly crass-sounding. But what happens to people who live more solitary lives, when they need help? Such thoughts went through my mind. Life trades. Choices.

There was some thought hovering at the periphery of my mind, though, some desire to have lived more fully these past decades. Though I wasn't sure what the actual enacting of that would have required. Maybe Martha needed to remember to drink more wine. Though she would have to tie a string to my finger to remind me. Where was Mary with the bottle? Keeping it to herself, still in some doorway?

The last full day of the festival, we went to another little restaurant, parked in the handicapped spot out front, and went in to order salad and something else. I remembered only the salad because we'd been advised of the treacheries of lettuce. Marty had, to that point, not choked on anything. But we were talking—what about?—and suddenly his face changed. His eyes watered—tears, I thought. He got up and went to the washroom, and then emerged some minutes later. He'd been struggling to breathe, I realized. He sat, catching his breath as much as he could. He stared at me, hard, and I could see fear. "Lettuce," he said. So the lettuce had caught in his throat. Such innocuous little bits of green nothing. We didn't sit for long. We got up, left the uneaten food, left the restaurant. People were looking at us; I remember faces as we passed to the door. Somehow Marty's movement to the washroom, and now our movement out, seemed out of keeping with the relaxed conversation and laughter and the comfort of the food, as others found it. Even the staff seemed irritated. Or was all that just some sensing of who-knows-what on my part? Did Marty's shadows show? Could that be felt on some level?

Later, he said he now needed to focus the entire time he was eating anything, he needed to be conscious of every chew and swallow. It made for silent meals. Food lost its pleasure and meals became a time of anxiety.

There was some feeling in me about all this that later I recognized as my "tank over the horizon" feeling. Something bearing down on us, that would happily pass right over and crush, if we didn't get the hell out of the way. Really, there was no getting out of the way. It just munched on. Mulched.

In my journal, on Whidbey, I scribbled a note: *I miss simple happiness.*

The sense of the oncoming tank felt to be a descent into some lowland. Would I have the strength I needed? I tried to hold to the thread of thought that I'd had the strength to date. There was no reason to think I wouldn't in future. I'd found it so far. But would that continue? Would strength materialize as I needed it? What if it didn't... *what if it didn't?*

When I followed Marty out of the restaurant that day, I wanted to stop. I wanted to find a place to sit and bawl. A foxhole. But we continued to the car, got in, drove to the B&B.

I needed to be alone, away from him, to let grief pour, and do its ugly and necessary thing. But as time passed, days and weeks, he needed me to be with him more and more. The burden grew, not to allow him to see the grieving process in me. Or to see enough to know I cared. How much did he need to see? How much did I need to let him see? How much did I need to hide? I didn't know the answers. What might be an answer could change, moment to moment.

41.

Five
Over Par

Using a golf cart
as never before
he plays five over
from the green tees
—tees closest to the fairway—
and is excited
and tells me

"You had a green tea game"
I say

He laughs

42.

Honk

CANADA GEESE WENT by, in the fall fog overhead, and I wondered if I would still have a husband when they returned.

The Archie Bunker chair—how I thought about the recliner with projectile capacity—was arriving Monday. I dreaded it. The Ice Bucket Challenge in the summer of 2014 had raised enough money to create warehouses of equipment for people living with ALS; the Archie chair was a part of that.

We had a last evening together on the couch, before the chair came. It was velvety and way too of the eighties in all its burgundyness. But I had a ten-minute nap in it, and damn, it was comfortable. Then it was Monday night, and we were firing up the television for an evening of *Downton Abbey*, and Marty asked if I'd like for him to sit next to me. I said yes, but that he also needed to be comfortable. It was his decision.

He chose the chair, and sat in it on the other side of the room. Somehow, anticipating the pending arrival of the chair over the weekend had allowed me—somewhat—to prepare for that moment. But it was still a moment. His choice hurt, but it was a necessary hurt, I reminded myself. Its purpose wasn't my pain. But the spot beside me on the couch was there, a most empty place.

The following evening, I thought to pull around the couch so that I could watch the television, and face him, too. But was so aware of the space between us.

43.

October Heartburn

I'D NEVER HAD pain like that. I panicked, wondered (warning: more irrational thinking ahead) if it was possible I had thyroid cancer, or something wrong with my neck. It felt as if there was something pushing both up and down. My jaw was aching. Sternum feeling stony. There was a sense of choking—though, given Marty's reality, I was loath to use that term. In my mind, I tried out the word "discomfort."

I'd been reading Joan Didion's *The Year of Magical Thinking*, in which she noted how common it was for a grieving person to experience earaches and infections—from the gathering of unshed tears. But I hadn't yet connected her words with my reality.

The feeling was so intense, I lay down. Which left me feeling silly. Tried to nap to make sense of the lying down. Thoughts imploded. Finally started to cry, and did so. Hard.

The pain went away. I realized then that it was indeed the physical *thing* of tears.

It was a bit unnerving, having read about it, assumed it meant others. Not me.

The ways the body can betray. The ways the body can nourish.

44.

Fundraising

MONEY CAME INTO our lives.

It began with the trickle—which sped then slowed and then sped again—of online fundraising.

It came in other ways too. Our friends, led by John D, events coordinator by profession as well as musician, put together a "Party for Marty" that rocked our little town. The fire marshal turned a blind eye to how many tickets we sold, and a number of bands played, and hundreds of items were donated to a silent auction. Friends worked in the bar, made food, decorated. Hours went into it. It was overwhelming. The sense of generosity and love was palpable, and pushed against the sad.

But there were other moments of giving, too. People would quietly hand off an envelope to him, and because Marty would be easily overcome with emotion at such moments, he took to coming home, and handing the envelopes to me to open. One stands out because it followed a wave of others, handed both to me as well as him, and elicited a particular emotional reaction from me—one that stymied and literally knocked me down. Amazing how the physical reaction mirrored the internal. Would I ever get used to this?

This envelope was given to him by someone at the golf course, who said that a person—anonymous—had handed it to him, and he was passing it along. Marty handed it to me, still sealed, and with his name typed on the outside. Someone did not want their handwriting recognized.

I took it upstairs, knowing that if I opened yet another of these in front of him, it would bring on more tears.

Upstairs, in front of the dresser drawer in which I kept this money, I opened the envelope: ten crisp browns—a thousand dollars.

There was still cash left from the barbershop fundraising. I tucked in the bills, alongside my underwear, thinking, *No one will go in here...*

I walked out of the room, started down the hallway, felt suddenly limp, and had to stand over the nearby laundry machines. I had an urge that was so big: an urge to return the money. All of it. To somehow track down every person who'd had a haircut that day at Billie's Barbershop, and to go to the golf course and *demand* to know the name of Anonymous, to hand over the bills and say, "Take it! Take it back! Take back the bathroom shower. We'll take it all apart, return it to what it was. Bring back the guitar students traipsing in and out of the house. Waiting in the bench in the carport under that clock that had hung forever on the wall, with parents picking them up on the driveway. Even bring back those parents who pissed me off by sitting in the driveway running their engines while waiting for a student. (If they want to run their engine, I'll say nothing ever again.)"

It had something to do with the anonymity. That was what made it impossible to return; as long as I didn't know where it was coming from, I couldn't return it. Somehow, in my mind this made the need for the funds more concrete. I realized that in my battling of hope and acceptance, the hope that a miracle would happen—and with that, a happiness in returning the money—was thwarted by acceptance: take the money, there will be no reason to return it, and be grateful.

Which I was. So grateful in so many moments and later days. But that moment filled with the desire to return the money. The *need* to return the money. And the hopelessness of knowing it wouldn't be. I was being utterly irrational, and knew it. But that did not change the irrational thing.

I wished I were a dreamer. A silly little dreamer.

MONTHS AFTER MARTY passed away, Ole asked if we would be putting the downstairs bathroom back to what it had been. Even as I was amazed that he didn't see the impossibility in this, there was something oddly heartening in how he thought it could happen. I was not the only one to have had this thought go through their mind. If we could all—all of us king's horses and men—just put it back to how it was.

45.

Team 4

IN LATE OCTOBER, there was a leak in the roof. Rain came in through the fan in the bathroom, dripping onto the toilet seat below. I awoke to the sound of the drip. It was too early to get up, and I valued every minute of Marty's sleep. He needed it. So I wrapped a towel over the toilet seat and closed the bathroom door, hoping to muffle the sound, glad for once for the earbud caught in his ear, blocking out the world. I got dressed quietly, and went to find a tarp and pony clips and rope. Climbed onto the roof from the upstairs deck, and set about covering the fan hood and surrounding area. Cursed the rain. Cursed the mistake in accepting the lowest-bid roofers as we'd done just a couple of years before. But maybe it wasn't them; maybe it was general laziness about upkeep. I didn't want to be out on the roof, playing roofer-mom. Even though it was a role I was not unused to, if I was honest about it. But at least there'd been a time when I could say, "Can you go out and look at the roof?" Could even promise there might be something in it for him if he did.

Martha, in the rain, tarping it up.

46.

Inside Out

Olivia takes family photos
and later Marty starts
to take off his purple and white golf shirt

Sudden anger
tense, ALS-sputtering, close to tears
"I wore this all day," he gasps. "No one told me
it was inside out"

I'd noticed
twice
But such work to take clothing off
and on   was hardly noticeable I'd thought
talked myself out
of saying anything about it

mistake

47.

Late Fall

IT WAS THE end of October, and I noted how when I pressed my face into Marty's back, it felt different. I couldn't find the easy place for my cheek behind his shoulder blade, as I used to. Or my forehead, or any part really. We used to tuck together so nicely, and now didn't. His back was new, changed, narrowed. It pushed me away. I began not to seek it out, as the pushing away hurt. Then came the night when I wrapped an arm around him, and he pushed my arm away, and told me he couldn't breathe when my arm was around him. Asked me not to do that. From that point on, I didn't.

Pieces go. We go in pieces, if we don't go all at once, it seems. We grieve in pieces, too.

But I managed to get through October without wiping September off the erasable calendar. Not so many years before, I did a year in an education program, a year that was so ugly-busy that it became a daily ritual—evening—to swipe a thick red marker across each day as it passed. There was satisfaction to that at first. But as months passed, and the evening red swipe continued, there began to feel something intrinsically wrong about the motion, the act, the results, of entire calendar pages being collections of red swipes, so that weeks and months became nothing more than a half dozen red lines, gone. Days shouldn't be counted, or discounted, like this, I remembered thinking. So it was a reward, at the close of that October, to realize I was not counting days thus. I was choosing to create a disconnect between the calendar and the reality of daytimes and nights, and their passing. A calendar is an arbitrary thing.

A day is each its own.

48.

Halloween Morning

Marty manages to cook an omelette with blue cheese
I have to open the coconut oil. I have to flip the
omelette. We forget the pepper. I decide it's time
to email the program chair at work, and let him know
I need to stop working
and I won't be able to teach in January

I try to remember the moment I decided to accept
this. And can't
Was it that Monday when I could not remove myself
from the couch on the deck?
Is acceptance the same as lack-of-hope?
is not-fighting giving up?

49

November Concert

MARTY'S SUMMER ROCK School always culminated in a celebration of sorts, a fall concert at the local recreation centre. This year followed tradition, except for the extra tears and hugs from the young students. Marty couldn't take the stairs up to the stage, so he directed from sitting below, with older students taking on leading roles as MC and stage manager. At the end of the night, he was trying to say something that I could not understand. He grew agitated, pushing my hand away, pushing at me, coming to a wobbly stand and motioning to a student to come closer, to listen. I realized he was trying to say that the closing band on stage had forgotten to perform a song in their set. But they hadn't. "They've done their four," I said. "They have?" he asked, perplexed.

At the end of the night, back home, that question came up again. "What is going to become of me? I'm just going to wither away, aren't I?" I put an arm around him as if that would stop all withering. "I don't want to wither away," he said, and then repeated it. "I know," I said. "I know." I'd already reassured him that we would take care of him, here at home, that was a promise. He would not wither away with strangers in an institution. But all I could do was to acknowledge these words; I couldn't change anything in any real way—at least, not in any way that would alter or deter the withering. And if he wouldn't share what else was in his mind, I couldn't speak to it. "We will always love you." That I could say with conviction.

50

Prayer for Christmas

AS THE WEATHER got colder, I found myself stepping out of doors. At first, I didn't really notice it consciously. I just had to be outdoors. Toes in the grass at end of summer, heavy robe on for early fall mornings while coffee brewed, sweater on as the weather chilled in October. I thought that I wanted to prolong the summer. But I also realized, as the weeks began to pass and speed up even, that going outside of the four walls of the house seemed to allow me to breathe a bit more easily. This realization was slow.

One day it hit me: I remembered my cousin, widowed suddenly at the age of fifty, and mentioning how she found herself outdoors, *had* to be outdoors. Though it was midwinter when she lost her spouse.

Midwinter. I dreaded it. We were going to make it through Christmas, I told myself. Family was coming from afar. We will have fun. We will. *Just get us through Christmas. Just let Marty eat at the big table with the family, all together. Turkey and all. No choking. Please no choking. One last Christmas dinner. Please.*

51.

Reach

I reach into the fridge for some supplement
Wonder if there is anything else at all that we could be
doing
The thought is always there, always torturing. Even
though I know, I know
IknowIknowIknow there is
nothing

52.

Snake Oil

EARLY ON, MARTY began to take liquid magnesium to help him sleep (there is documentation of low levels of magnesium and calcium in people with ALS), and I ordered a particular brand from one of our two local health food stores, a funky little orange house situated by the slough that ran behind one of the main streets. I'd always liked to walk into the place—it smelled good, and most of the employees were friendly and knowledgeable. I ordered a case of bottles after Marty finished the first one. I thought it was a good product, and it did indeed seem to help him sleep. The owner, noting my purchase, asked if I'd be interested in writing a product review, and said she'd be happy to give me an extra bottle. It wouldn't take me long. Someone might find it useful, I thought.

So I wrote a brief blurb, noted the illness, the need to sleep, and the fact that it did seem to aid. Everything about ALS is so incremental, that any bit of respite is just that. I thought the blurb did the trick and emailed it to the owner. Back it came. Along with an example of the "sort of thing I am looking for." Something raving and enthusiastic for wonder product, capable of The Cure.

"I can't write that," I wrote back. "That's just not true. We're talking ALS here," I reminded her, almost adding, "You know... the disease that is beyond Stephen Hawking!"

Well, then, she didn't feel she could offer me a free bottle, was her response.

It wasn't about the bottle, I let her know. Really, did she have to add that? Then—from somewhere in me—came a few bluntly worded thoughts about why health food folks can find accusations of snake oil peddler thrown at them. She had one of the nice employees email me an apology. I was glad there were two stores in town.

53.

Junk Mail

ONE DAY I put the mail on the kitchen table—usual bills and flyers, and an envelope addressed to "Guitar Marty"—and got on with my day. I'd now trained myself not to hand over any mail to Marty, and he hadn't paid much attention to the mail for a while. So I was surprised to see this envelope later, in his hands. He'd opened it, and appeared to be stymied. I recognized it instantly as junk mail, albeit with a name on it. I should have thrown it out. A missed step.

I looked closely, and guessed that it came from someone connected with his work of teaching music in the local schools, though that seemed to be a bit of a stretch: it was a pizza order form, for classroom pizza. But advertisers can be desperate people with a quota to fill.

The look on his face, though, that he was not understanding what this was, and was not capable of such, broke my heart. Who were these idiots who addressed this envelope and sent it out? (Though my rational brain questioned how they could possibly know. The conversations between these two parts of my brain made me want to shout.)

I explained to him, and at the same time, squelched my mounting panic that I must do this, that this was our reality. I explained junk mail to my husband, who in the past had explained to me how computers work.

54.

Makes My Day

I return home from teaching, mid-afternoon, and pull
into the driveway. My brain plays that trick on me, a
flash
image: Marty, coming out of his studio, through the
carport door, saying, "Honey!"
Sadness floods me, rises, carries flotsam
Or begins to

The door opens and there he is. Shaky, but there
"Honey!"

55.

To Seize

I STRUGGLED TO describe this disease, even to myself. There was both an appalling silence about it—it does silence the person who lives with it—and a violence. A violence made more fearsome by the silence. I wrote a piece in my journal, an attempt to capture the sense of the thing:

They move in under the feather quilt, summer light. He is asleep in seconds, but it takes her a while longer before she drifts off. She likes this piece of time, the sense of being alone yet not. The stirring of sound in her wind chimes out the patio door. That is open too. It is a summer evening, perfect in every way. She falls asleep at last.

She comes to, more than awakening. It is dark, the moon has moved away. Run away maybe. It is so dark, she realizes, even as she feels the loud and sudden silence. Is that what woke her? She reaches beside her to feel for him. But she can't move. The strange sensation of movement in her arm is just that—strange. It is not movement. An amputee thing. Ghost arm—she hears the phrase in her head.

Then a still silence. What she hears is not a sound. It's an awareness. From the not-moving fingers in her hand, through her wrist, elbow, arm, she feels numbness. There is something here, in her bed, something with her husband. It is causing the numb in her, the inability to move. She tries to say his name. She hears it in her head, but she can't speak it. Then, clearly, she knows he can't speak either. She just knows. He can't move. This thing, this numbing thing is acting on him. Raping him, is what she thinks. She doesn't have this thought with her mind; the thought penetrates from her centre, from deep behind her navel, where the word rape lives in women, in a cave with a heavy stone across its door, a stone that should not be moved.

This beside her is something silent and violent. More than anything she wants sound and movement, to know what it is that she is living with. But there's just this darkness. There is pain here. Her husband's pain leaks into her. She can feel it, an acid through her skin, into her bones.

There is a withdrawal, cold air sudden and next to her, and somehow this numbing being has managed to take up her husband in its arms—because she knows it has arms—and is carrying him away toward the open patio door. There is the darkest silhouette there, black on black. She is trying to think his name, and the word stop, but nothing comes from her, not even a breath, and then there is just the rectangle of doorway, a lighter dark. How strong is this thing that it can pick up, still so silent, and carry away. She remembers then that the Latin word from which we've grown 'rape' means to seize, and to carry away. Her mind tells her these thoughts are absurd, absurd that she can even think about word origin at this time. But the banality of the nature of the thought is a preserver to hold on to. Words.

What were her last words to him. What were his words to her? Was there anything sustaining in those words? Why does she feel she'll never see him again, never hear his voice, never feel his arms around her? She can't put hers around him. How can this be?

She lies in the darkness unable to move, stricken.

56.

Team 5

EARLY NOVEMBER, AND one member of his golf foursome, John M, brought home two boxes of belongings from
Marty's locker at the golf club. The boxes sat in the front
entranceway. Marty was in his studio at the time. John grew
teary bringing them in. He left, and I stood there feeling the
goodbye in those boxes. The golf season had come to an end
weeks ago. I was aware—I was so aware—that the seasons
were with us. That Marty had been able to play through the
beautiful and forgiving summer months, that as the disease
took over, the summer wound down and retreated grace-
fully, that as fall encroached there was a natural loss. Could
I say that? There was nothing natural about this. Yet everything, too. How was that? But winter was coming, and here
were the boxes, and now I had to do something with them.

I had to hide them, and hope he didn't come out of his
studio as I was doing that.

The storeroom—an unfinished space that included
our woodpile, tool bench, musical gear, and sports equipment—was right off the studio. I made room on a high
shelf, somewhere he would not notice. I sneaked in the first

box. No sound from the studio; what did he do in there, all day? Although he had not taught a student since mid-August, he liked to spend the bulk of his day there, as he had for so many years. He felt useful in that room. Right now, his project was to take family videos, and render them into something we would be able to locate and watch in the future. In the family, he had been the IT person. He may not have been the handyman, but he had taken care of family archives—photography and video. For the kids' sports teams, he was the go-to guy for team videos, which he'd create and share at the end-of-season wrap parties and barbecues. Hockey and baseball parents would be so pleased.

I sneaked in the second box, and caught sight of the things in the boxes: golf balls, gloves of wrinkled bits of leather, no doubt beyond use, but I was loath to throw away. There were also old rain pants, still with dried mud and, in a box corner, ageing packets of hand and feet warmers.

The sorting was a job for Martha; I pushed the boxes back as far as I could, hoping Marty never spotted them. Ole could go through them someday. I cried. Put away the ladder, left the room.

I was tired of hiding.

57

Slowed to
the Slowest

I eat my breakfast like a new mother
who will be called in to nurse
at any moment: hardly
chewing, swallowing dry
The person across the table from me is
mindful of every push
of his tongue, every motion
of his jaws

I slow
The teacher in me wonders what
it would be, every lesson, every class, if every
learner—and the teacher—
slowed to the slowest in the room; what would we
notice? What would change?
Or would we be filled with
impatience? I clear the table, and Marty comments:
"You do that so easily"
"I don't take it for granted," I say, feeling
trucked-over exhausted

I tell him, "Sometimes, when I'm
in dance class, I look in the mirror, and
I'm amazed I can do
anything"

58.

Wind Chimes

FOR WEEKS, EMMETT considered it his job to assist his dad up the stairs to our room at bedtime. No matter what he was doing, he'd be on the spot. But into November it became not only difficult, but rather frightening to support his dad's weight, and we worried he might topple backward.

One night, Marty didn't want to have to climb the stairs at all. So much so that he proposed to sleep alone downstairs. I persuaded him to do one more night upstairs in the room we'd shared for sixteen years, one more night to bring closure. To ponder what it is to walk down a hallway, and climb down stairs one last time under one's own roof. What is it to know that an entire part of your home will no longer be part of your life?

Not sure why I needed that night, and he appeared not to. But he did humour me with one more trip up the stairs.

In the morning, the last morning, light came through the curtain.

I listened to the wind chimes outside the patio doors off the bedroom. Last time, I thought, with us lying there.

I'd always loved the sounds of chimes, but Marty hadn't. He could tolerate them. Oddly, it wasn't until that last couple of years that I'd bought some for myself to enjoy; inherent in loving someone—I believe—should be the room to stretch and differentiate. If I'd purchased them before then, when we drifted apart, they would have been a point of antagonism.

So we'd lived with them through some windy Novembers and Marches, and when wind gusted, I would throw on a robe in the middle of the night and take down their enthusiastic peal, and re-hang them for another night of lighter musical fare. We built some modicum of acceptance and knowing when enough was enough.

Now November wind rattled them again—last time—and rain slashed the windows. Last time. March seemed a long ways off.

Was this healthy on my part—this refrain of *last time* sounding though me? I didn't know. I only knew I needed to slow time as much as possible, and needed the one extra night. To pause. Some Mary gesture—to sit and listen.

Then time again to move with change.

59.

Team 6

I HADN'T BEEN to a yoga class since some time in the summer. I'd had a four-year-long practice, to that point, and was so grateful to have developed that piece in my life. So even when days passed without, I could feel in my mind the restorative power.

I had a handful of DVDs from my sister-in-law, and a friend had left one in the mailbox, a DVD with several twenty-minute routines. Twenty minutes was perfect, I discovered. Even that was interrupted some days. Some days I did not do even ten minutes, had to pause it, and returned to it hours later. But there was a day in November when I pulled out the one-hour DVD—*Yoga Warrior*, it was called—pulled on my yoga pants, rolled out my mat, and managed to get through from beginning to end.

I wanted to tell someone, "I did it! An hour!"

I couldn't. I couldn't go into the studio, to find Marty picking over his keyboard, to share with him that my body still moved in all the ways I wanted it to. I had to keep it to myself. Why was a goal met less so when it was not shared?

60.

Downstairs

FIRST NIGHT DOWNSTAIRS. How very odd to have set up a bed in Marty's work studio. Hanging guitars filled the wall, and so many computer and equipment lights made the room look like a miniature airport at night. How would I ever sleep? There was the quiet whir of electronics, a sound I can't stand. (Give me battling, bellowing wind chimes any night.) For Marty to be closer to the door and the bathroom, we changed sides of the bed. I'd tried to convince him that a urinal might be a good idea, but he'd resisted. I hadn't pushed too hard; the changes were so many, the relinquishing so great. Outside the "bedroom" door, with the smell of fresh plywood, was the ramp that my brother and father had built to the new bathroom.

In the middle of the night, Marty got up. Hard to say if it was the unfamiliar side, or what exactly, but the next thing I heard was the sound of him falling on the plywood floor. A sound that echoed through my gut. Moaning followed. My first thought—after my heart folded in on itself—was that there was something to trip over, but no. Except possibly his own foot dragging. I fought the feeling that I could have done something to prevent this. With ALS, when a person falls, they can't catch themselves. He had bruises down the side of his body. Somehow his head had only a small cut at the temple. I was shaking as I helped him to the bathroom. I said nothing about a urinal, but once I had him back in bed, I went to the storeroom to fetch the walker that a neighbour had loaned us some weeks before. We hadn't yet used it inside the house. That night, there were three more trips to the toilet, all with the walker.

I didn't realize the following day was Remembrance Day until I showed up at the small pharmacy under Dr. K's office, with its blinds drawn and a closed sign in the window. I wanted to cry when I saw it. Usually Remembrance Day finds me at the cenotaph, or at least running out to the deck to see the small airplanes fly overhead around noon at the ceremony's close. I'd completely forgotten the day. Now it was the impediment to getting what I most needed.

I peered through the window. As if that would help. Saw a woman in the back room, and had immediate knowledge of what had brought her here; she was doing that happy puttering in the worksite on a holiday—the luxury of Uninterrupted Time.

I knocked. Tentatively. She came to the door, and opened it. As soon as I began with, "My husband has ALS, and—" I didn't even get to the "need a urinal" bit, and she opened it wide. I went home with the teal urinal that looked like a beekeeper's smoke-blower (as Dr. K pointed out), and Marty's reluctance was won over after one use. Bonus: He got back his side of the bed, once toilet proximity was not an issue. Normalcy.

USUALLY WE HUNG our Christmas lights on Remembrance Day. When it comes and goes without, there is something amiss. It almost came and went.

The phone rang that morning, with my sister-in-law, then a friend, followed by another, Louise. I talked with each, short conversations, then had to hang up, talked out.

It didn't feel right to let this Christmas-light tradition go. When Marty napped, I slipped outside and wrapped a couple of strands around the weeping birch out front. As I stood back to take a look, it occurred to me that I could have asked Louise to come and help. She lived just down the street, and we could have sipped coffee between stringing strands. But the thought of having to talk—just the thought—wore me out. It soothed me to hang the lights in silence, with some ambiguous holiday song humming in my head. Maybe "I'll Be Home for Christmas" with its war-era closing line.

I discovered a few overlooked bulbs of garlic out in a vegetable bed, raked leaves in the garden, revelled in the silence. I needed hours and hours of silence that almost never happened.

A time of remembrance. Not of the past, but of a moment just then.

WHEN I CALLED the man who had done the tile in the bathroom, to see if he could suggest someone or help to add a handrail to the shower, when I explained that Marty had fallen the night before, and that the slipperiness of the bathroom was my immediate concern, he showed up. He put the handrail in that afternoon.

I asked him how much I owed.

He said, "Merry Christmas."

61.

Shoe Shelf

I EMPTIED A shelf of shoes in the storeroom. Most of them were too heavy for Marty to wear. Only one particular pair was now comfortable, the lightest of summer shoes; anything else required too much effort. I put the other shoes in a corner. We needed the shelf as a bedside table in the new bedroom.

"I need my shoe shelf," he said, when he saw me moving it. The words were slurred, fuzzy. But there was also a vagueness to his tone, as if they weren't what he meant to say, as if there was some part of him that *knew* he didn't really need that shelf. Not for shoes.

They were words he would have said months ago if he'd seen me doing this; it was as if his brain could not keep up with his reality.

I started to say, "No you don't," but stopped. The "no" hung in the air. I added "not right now," as if there would be a "later." But we both knew.

How could I rein in my thoughts and my knowledge? Not for the first time, I wondered about how people without children would go through this. How do they motivate themselves?

How to twin the now and what's to come. Or how to do one, and then the other.

62.

Pieces

DEEP INTO FALL a number of elements came together. Or apart. Golf game over, Marty's ability to drive the car gone, bedroom downstairs, Big Chair in our lives. In spite of me finding a warm and light winter poncho for the borrowed wheelchair, he had no interest in going back outside. Except for the occasional trip to hospital, we were relegated to being inside the house.

I found this difficult, even as I struggled to make it to my two or three teaching sessions each week. I left the house as late as I could and returned as quickly as possible, and had teaching assistants or guests lecture for me often. I checked texts from home throughout the last bit of class time, and would receive messages that threw me into a panic. I did speak with the chair of the program about finding a replacement to complete the workshop class, and schedule this person to take over for the second half of class in January; I'd come to terms with the fact that I was going to need a full leave soon.

Some changes were pushed at us, and others we rode with in some way. At times, Marty initiated the changes.

So there came a day when I placed food on the small table that he used to eat from the Big Chair, expecting him to move the table into place as he had to that point. Instead, he stared at me, wordlessly asking me, expecting me, to move it.

I did, with an unsettled feeling. Did he need me to move that table? Or was he relinquishing something? If so, what? His autonomy, certainly. What else?

I felt servile in that moment, and there was a question in my mind about the necessity of the request. I had no problem with giving and helping, and being generally useful. But. There was a "but" in my mind. This smacked of not even being taken for granted, but being deliberately pushed, asked of. I moved the table, but wasn't happy about it.

When should someone give up? When should someone expect others to do for? How judgmental was I being? Should I have offered? Why was there a twinge within me of feeling badly that I hadn't offered? *Why* would I have offered? How to recognize when someone needs help. Yet if they ask for it, surely they need it. Where are all the lines between two people, in communication, miscommunication, expectations, helping, being helpless, understanding? I could go on. All these negotiables that occur through the day, some resulting in hurts, some in minor joys. Maybe it was nothing beyond asking for a table being moved, something he felt he needed just in that moment.

Big Things in relationships: a sense of being seen (do you *see* me?) and heard (do you understand what I'm saying? or at least *hear*?). Maybe it was just that.

But that undercurrent, a coming to pieces—at this point, I didn't so much as articulate this to myself—and I countered it with mental images I would run through my mind, to remind me of the man who shared my home, with his face that showed less and less of what he was feeling, and his slowed body. I would close my eyes and envision his expressions of happiness in our past, his smile, his quick laugh. The way he'd walked, or set his hands on his hips while listening to someone speak, the way he held a cigarette, or crossed his legs while we sat at the fire. The way he played guitar. As the months passed, I ran such images through my mind several times a day. Remembered who he'd been. Who he still was, now trapped.

When friends and acquaintances, even relatives, learned that I was working on a piece about caregiving, a surprising number of them asked me this: "How do you not hate the person you are caregiving?" Maybe they meant words like "not resent." But what came out was the word "hate."

The first thing that came to mind in answer to this were those mental images. The images helped stave off the negatives. They served to soften my heart. Softer things might not be so brittle, might not break so easily.

I AWOKE IN the middle of the night to find my husband's neck and back wet with tears, lying beside me. He must have been lying on his back, and rolled away. Which was not easy.

I rubbed his back until his breathing settled to deep sleep.

I'd been in early motherhood mode through all these months, awakening immediately every time he stirred, or left the room to go pee. I hadn't been in that mode for so long, for so many years, all so passed now, yet here I was again. No thought put into it even—just old pattern emerging from shadows.

The next teaching day—one of my last—I made my way through rain to the university, begrudging every minute in the car, yet glad to have a car, glad to shorten the trip and time as much as possible. The car gave me a sense of control I didn't have using transit.

I parked at the parkade nearest to my office, and hurried in. When I did go to work, the entire time felt to be rushed, a sense of in and out. No time to really think about what I was doing; I'd taught for so long that much could go on autopilot. But it wasn't the way I liked to work with young people learning, and I was left feeling guilty both to students and to myself.

I walked across the concrete slabs of the courtyard between the Buchanan buildings, where I've been both student and teacher off and on for decades. A path that had felt familiar and even familial just one year ago when I'd returned to teach after a half dozen years spent elsewhere. One year ago, I'd been fifty years old, with a marriage that gave a sense of purpose and peace, and with the job I'd wanted for too long. With enlivening, striving students. After years of struggling to make ends meet, growing my sons, growing my self—suddenly all the pieces seemed to have come together. Three weeks before Marty's diagnosis, I'd told him how much I loved my fiftieth year, how it could go on without end, and I'd be happy.

I crossed that courtyard, grey and wet, and felt sudden breath-stopping deep red panic, followed by an urgent need just to be home. I continued to my class, struggling to quash that feeling, and taught the two hundred plus students. I finished, prepared to leave, and checked my phone.

A text from Marty let me know he couldn't find his teeth.

He hadn't had his own teeth in decades. They'd been weakened by scarlet fever as a toddler, and removed in his mid-teens. (There goes the Internet theory of the effects of dental fillings as a cause of ALS.) I knew that without his teeth he couldn't eat, and what was left of his ability to talk would be further compromised.

I arrived home and found the dentures under the dresser. They'd fallen, and in trying to find them, he'd knocked them farther under, almost to the wall. He couldn't bend over to see, and risk himself falling. He would not be able to get back up; that was beyond him at that point. He was almost in tears when I arrived, and hungry. Embarrassed with his need.

I said nothing about how I'd come home, driving so fast that scenarios of being stopped and questioned played through my mind. Would a cop believe me if I explained why I was thirty kilometres over the limit? Or why I cut across that person in the BMW? *Just let me get home safely. Quickly.*

Through these months there was a constant sense of urgency to my gut, my joints, my muscles. Except for when I was asleep—though judging by how I felt on waking, maybe not even then. I was in a dreamless state for the most part, and my own teeth hurt from indefinable jaw pain. A week later, I went in to discuss with the dentist, and he ground down a few edges, said they weren't sitting right. Months later, he removed a molar in pieces, cracked in two from clenching.

63.

Walking After Midnight

EMMETT IS PLANNING an evening walk, as he often does. Marty and I are readying for bed; that can take an hour, and we go to bed so so early.

Somehow though, I pick up on a different energy from Emmett. I hear him go out. I lie there, feeling anxious about my youngest. It hasn't been a good day.

Finally, I text him, thank him for all the help he gives his dad, tell him to enjoy his walk. *Someday I will join you again out there in the moonlight.*

Later, he returns. Through the walls I can hear him singing.

All is right with the world, just then.

64.

Band-Aid

I WOKE UP on a day in mid-November, trying to remember if I was a kid who liked the band-aid ripped off, or pulled away slowly, thinking that "slowly" could somehow side-step pain.

I used to prefer the latter, was the conclusion I came to. How did this connect with just wanting to remove the skin I was in?

THAT SAME MORNING, Marty decided he needed the walker to get around the house. Again, our world shifted.

I did the usual preparation for breakfast while he was in the bathroom. I set out the denture fixative. It had taken more than a few days to get the amount right. I applied it with a toothpick. Couldn't be too much or too little. But that day, Marty decided to rinse his teeth, and then he set the lower plate on the seat of the walker, pushing into the kitchen, rinsing it, and returning to the table with the teeth again on the seat. It struck me as both funny-sad and as an act that embodied dignity.

This is us, I thought. This is us now. Strange how a camera seemed to move out of my head, trying to gain a perspective on this. Looking back, looking down. Inside.

Later, after my own shower, I caught sight of my body in the mirror. It was changing. My thighs were heavier. My upper arms were loosening with the missing hours of yoga. It was a body being shaped by stress. My face was odd in some way I couldn't articulate. But someone would volunteer to do that for me—that was a given. I knew I didn't feel healthy anymore. I was sluggish. Less energetic even though I used more strength than I ever had in my life, just in what I did hour by hour. But I was less flexible, less nimble. I missed moving, and moving quickly, and vigorous lovemaking. Maybe that, more than anything.

In the middle of one night, Marty reached for me and pulled me into him with a cry, and with arms that felt to be from the past, so strong. At first I thought it was a dream, and then realized I was awake. But he didn't seem to be. After just a moment of holding, he released me, sighed, and was most soundly asleep. Leaving me wide awake and wondering.

Somehow sex felt of late to be more about resolution and getting off instead of lovemaking. Yet how could that be at this point in time? Was it about dying, and such focus on the body? I wondered. But my mind didn't sit there too long. There was something so normalizing about sex—even slowed sex—that made it feel necessary. For as long as it could be. Such as it was.

I couldn't stop my mind from roving to the future, skirting it, poking at... something. *Loneliness*, I realized. I pulled my mind back. *No.*

Later, going to sleep at the end of another day, I thought of the good things in the day: today Marty took some pleasure in his food; asked for pasta with clam sauce; we found a new series, *The Knick*, and enjoyed watching it; he didn't take a tumble; and something funny was said and laughed at, but I couldn't remember what it was.

It'll come to me, I scribbled in my journal.

I remembered: I pinched his bottom, as he walker-ed out of the kitchen into his studio, and he quirked something like his old grin at me. That was noteworthy.

65.

Headaches

Headaches become a Thing
apparently part of ALS
too much carbon dioxide
in the system. There is talk
about a bipap machine, and another
machine, something that belongs
in a dentist's office, to suck out excess phlegm. And a
nebulizer
with saline mist to breathe. And more. Machines
when I think about them
and using them, and manuals, and breaking down, and
noises in the night—
scare me

66.

The Bathroom Escaping

THE FASCINATION WITH body function that is a hallmark
of new motherhood, even for those who pride themselves
on being beyond or above such, had once again become a
part of my life. Not something I planned. With it came the
inevitable scrutiny of bathrooms.

Even in the early stages, with the onset of symptoms, I
became aware of how our immediate world of home was
changing.

There was a window in the ensuite bathroom, and immediately outside this window was a weeping birch. In the summer,
the glass was filled with delicious little green leaves. In the
fall, the leaves were rattly orange. In the winter, when the
branches were bare, I put up a curtain of mulberry organza.

Once the window was in place, spiders became part of
the bathroom-scape. It had been Marty's household task
to clean that room, and with the *thing* he had for spiders,
it was his routine to vacuum the poor things—except he
always left the one with the busiest web, the most captures.
I didn't want to hear about the vacuuming bit. I'd remind

him that as much as he feared spiders, he loathed mosquitoes more, zzzz-ing in the night and sucking his blood.

At the time of renovating that downstairs bathroom, our little en suite began to take on a feel of the forsaken.

I often ask writing students to consider the difference between a character *knowing* something is about to happen versus *not knowing*. Tension comes, I believe, from knowing. Consider the difference between walking into a house, when you feel certain that someone is lying in wait for you, versus walking in and being surprised when someone leaps out at you. True, the leaping out might be enough to cause you to pee yourself, and the adrenalin will overwhelm. But if you walk into a silent house, in the middle of the night, lights out, and you know someone is *there*, and you begin to imagine you hear his breathing, and you can hear your own heartbeat, and everything inside you is churning and knotting... that is tension.

So maybe the analogy falls apart, as it is the *bathroom* I'm talking about. But maybe the analogy works for ALS itself. Or the difference between a terminal diagnosis and any diagnosis with some shred of hope. With the terminal diagnosis, something is always *there*, waiting.

This little room—smallest in the house—was now left behind, with our move to sleeping downstairs. I still used it as a shower once in a while, but every time I did, I was reminded that at some point I would return to it as *my* bathroom—and when I did, I would be a different person. Who, I didn't know.

For now, it was one of the few places I was alone.

Back in the time of the end of summer, late one morning when I could finally find time to shower, and Marty had gone golfing, I'd discovered a leaf from the weeping birch had wandered in through the open window, and was perched on the back of the toilet. I'd picked it up and tossed it back out.

Downstairs, in the new bathroom, the toilet had been put in place the third week of September, and at that point, Marty had begun to make only one daily trip upstairs, to bed. Thinking about it at that point—late November—and remembering how he'd wondered at my flurry of activity to renovate. Then he'd suddenly needed the renovation, needed not to haul himself up the stairs. He'd been grateful to have the new downstairs facilities... even as I was stunned that we needed them, and that we'd made it happen with family and neighbours pitching in.

There were many such moments, out-of-mind experiences, where something took me over, and I'd have to begin some process, or make a decision, or just *do* something. Then look back, and wonder: How did that happen?

Even in late September, the upstairs en suite window was still open. Again I found a birch leaf, not green, but gold and curled with dryness, on the back of the toilet. I went to toss it out the window, but instead held it in my hand. There was an insistence to this leaf. It was another piece, reminding me it was fall, and that the seasons were changing. This would be a last season. Another last season. I left the leaf on the back of the toilet, gold on white. In just that moment— to be repeated—I was ready for fall. Whatever that meant.

Now, late in November, the en suite was mine alone. It became—along with the car—my place to cry. No one could hear me. I could feel hot water sluicing over me, and that felt good because my body was beginning to ache at that point.

It was now also my job to clean that room, but I never seemed to have time for that. A quick swipe at the sink, swoop of a toilet brush. Dust and spiderwebs grew. I didn't vacuum spiders, so long as they stayed safely in their corners. Those ubiquitous leaves were in the corners, too, now. Even with window closed, and I didn't want to clean them out. I left the leaves. They reminded me that there was an outside world. If I couldn't go out to it, it would come in to me, and let me know, remind me, it would be ready for me to return. It would be waiting. Loving.

There was one extraordinarily tired morning, when I stood in the shower, with winter light through the window. I leaned against the wall, closed my eyes. All I wanted was the hot hot water, and the nothingness of it. I looked up to see the shadow of one long, thin-legged beauty who'd emerged from a corner, and was climbing delicately over the shampoo holder, drops of water falling, making her flinch, and still she travelled.

I let her be.

67.

Reverse

I have another dream
A young and favourite guitar student of Marty's, along
with her mother, are in a car
Marty is walking behind their car
With all the logic of dreams
The mother puts the car in reverse and begins to back
up—leaving me screaming for her attention and to Marty
to move, which of course he can't
I can't get there
in time. I'm of no use
I wake up

68.

Small Hours

IN THE LAST days of November, he awoke in the small hours of the morning gasping, and I pulled him up to sitting. I panicked—I was instantly awake—then slowed myself, and rubbed his back to calm both of us, reminding myself not to reach around him, not to hug. I moved from muttering "what happened" to silence. I analyzed later, and realized that fluffy pillows were a problem. His own pillow was that pricey thing we'd picked up in Portland, shaped with memory foam to support his neck. I figured he must have turned towards me, and my down-filled pillow got caught in his mouth. Until he couldn't breathe.

I've never been able to sleep on a flat pillow—the Romans came to mind, with their rocks, and about as comfortable. But I now had a note on my list of to-do: get rid of pillow. I found a thin lifeless pillow in one of the boys' beds and traded it for my fluff.

Not even two weeks later, the wee hours panic happened again, and I soothed him like an old pro—though inwardly in shock. Not for the first time, I worried that my calmness would send a message of a lack of care. Over breakfast, I asked him if my reaction was helpful, and he said, "Yes," with a serious tone. But still—

I hoped Martha didn't keep score, and feel she was victorious in some way. She was just doing her thing, that was all. I reminded her of that.

Mary had gone off to swing on her big one under the maple tree. Back and forth, like a kid, trying to touch the clouds with her bare feet, and seeming not to give a shit about all that needed to be done.

The to-do list grew.

69.

CBC in the Morning

has an interview with someone about right-to-die
that's all abuzz now with
changing laws—soon, they promise
we eat breakfast and listen and pretend
not to be listening

someone describing fears of dying choking
choking while eating
I can't turn it off
he won't let me

he is looking at me
That's what I'm afraid of, he says

—at least, that's what I think
he says

70.

Almost December

I CLEANED THE downstairs of the house and put up indoor Christmas lights. I needed the colour, the brightness. I found an old set of CDs, acoustic Christmas, and listened to one on the way to work. Only one week of one class was left. But the music was too slow, and made me sad. I had that feeling—never far away—of wanting to scratch my way out of my skin.

I turned it off and drove with silence instead.

I WENT THROUGH bills and paid. I'd now taken some of the fundraised money, cleaned up, consolidated debt into something manageable. Closed down credit cards I had no idea we had; obviously Marty's cognition had been affected longer than any of us knew. I discovered an entire second chequing account that some "advisor" at the local bank had opened, and was supposed to have closed down the original account, but somehow we'd been paying monthly insufficient funds penalties, and oh my, what a mess. It took hours on the phone to make it all go away. I suggested to the bank manager that they have an info session on dealing with baby boomers and neurological conditions; it was not limited to John Mann of Spirit of the West

I thought about the first book I ordered online to learn about this disease. It was a book published in the United States, and the final third of it was on how to negotiate insurance companies and claims. I remembered thinking how this was just not right—no one should have to do this when dealing with terminal illness.

It was time to work through disability forms, as discussed with our accountant. My gut was a mess. I wrestled with a feeling that trust was needed; trust that on some level, things would work out, whatever that meant. Well, maybe not work out... but work through. Somehow. I had to trust that. How would any of this ever make sense? What was it Vivienne had said outside the bakery that long-ago summer day? About someday this will make sense? She was wrong. This would not ever make sense or fall into some place.

I was stunned when, after mailing off the government disability forms December 17, I received a call from Victoria, home of government offices in the province, early afternoon on Christmas Eve, wanting to ascertain information so they could begin to process my request and paperwork immediately in the new year.

ALS forms were moved to the top of the pile, said the man on the other end.

71.

Teatime

My parents are coming for tea in the mid-afternoon
Early in the morning, Marty has discovered the day is
already rough
and thinks to take a marijuana capsule to calm. This is a
new point of exploration. He's acquired capsules, oil, some
edibles
different forms with which to experiment
Hours later, I receive a text
IM STONED
I check on him, tuck him into bed, wild-eyed
Tell Mom and Dad that today he'll be napping
through teatime

72.

Socks and Tree

ON MY WAY to the grocery store one day, I stopped at Mark's Work Wearhouse, and bought socks for everyone as Christmas stocking stuffers. I had in my mind to do more shopping, perhaps online or... the planning was vague. Imagination in short supply, with expiry day long passed. Somehow, the gift part of the holiday seemed so utterly unimportant.

What was important was that family was coming, dinner had to be tasty, and that we must have the annual music party as always, the Sunday before.

The tree, though. Now there was a question. With our vaulted ceiling, I tended to go somewhat over the top. Charlie Brown trees, with a mere handful of branches, were my tree of choice, but they had to be at least fifteen feet. This year, though, I mentioned the possibility of an artificial and was quickly shut down by Emmett. My reason, though, wasn't ease; it was my reluctance to have to deal with a dead thing at the end of the holiday. But then, I knew I'd enjoy a live tree at the outset of next year. *I may need that,* I thought.

My mother went with me, to the nearest tree lot, run by the Chung family for decades. My mother's van could hold a forest in it, and she did so love trees. One of the ageing Ms. Chungs followed us from afar as we poked at the trees. My mother and I took turns, holding up one and then another. I usually have a good eye—inherited from the carpenters in my family—to see exactly the height I need, but that day nothing looked right. I began to get the feeling I often do when shopping: *I just want to go home.* Then Ms. Chung moved in closer and began to hold up trees and run commentary.

I asked the woman to please leave us alone. I've never been comfortable doing such assertive actions, but I asked a second time too. I told her I needed to take my time. But she stayed right behind me, though she stopped holding up trees. I finally said that I really couldn't walk away with a huge tree, and could she *please* leave us alone to make a choice.

At that point all the trees looked horrible. No needles on branches. A yellowy colour. Enough stuff on top, but far-spread branches below. Or nothing on top—a single spindle that would bend over once the star went on. It began to feel like the hardest thing I'd done in days. Ridiculous. Still Ms. Chung wouldn't go. I told her this was a Christmas like no other, that it was a tough one, and I was having problems.

"Everyone has Christmas problems," she said, with a fucked-up half smile.

"No, this is a real problem," I said. Then I turned away, even though that left me facing the main street of our little town, and I started to cry. Mom gave me a good hug, and for once she didn't say anything about Jesus; I wholly felt her own care for me. I recovered.

I went over to look through some trees leaned against a fence, and my mother suggested the ones lying nearby. We pulled out a couple. The second one looked full, top full, branches nice, beautiful shade of green. Suddenly, all looked Good. Thirty-five dollars, chimed in Ms. Chung from afar. I carried it out. My mother chatted with Old Man Chung about his fish business.

They gave us each an orange. Mr. Chung said his father told him to do this years ago. I resolved to use my orange in Marty's morning drink when we returned home.

At home, I went to put the tree in a bucket, but asked my dad to do it because he needed to. He's always liked to pick up trees and do things with them.

73.

Christmas Eve

EARLY IN THE morning, and Ole was at the table, as was I, and Marty came along, stark naked, with his walker post-shower. I made a crack about a streaker. And Marty laughed, laughed harder, and the three of us laughed, and it was altogether a good moment, even though it ended in tears as he took his place in the big chair, ready for me to dress him. Dressing always had tears, a daily reminder of being unable to do the simplest. At times I imagined him as a little boy, excited about tying his own shoe for the first time, or I'd remember what it is to push a button through a buttonhole when one's fingers are tiny.

A few days later, the boys had a discussion about the nature of the walker progression across and through the living room. Ole had a tendency to deposit things —"put that anywhere," his dad always said to him. Now, as Marty pushed his way across the floor someone jumped up to move items out of his path. Over the holidays there were extras: a card table with a puzzle growing on it, games, boots, a hockey stick, extra pieces of outerwear clothing.

"It's like a video game," Emmett said. "Clearing things before Dad passes through the space."

Laughter gleaning.

74.

Rats

IN THE MORNING, I went into the storeroom for the potatoes. The potatoes were fine, but the bag of beets had a small
pile of bits of plastic and purple beside it. Nibblings. Rats.

We lived on a delta, rich farmland, bordered by river and
ocean. Rodents lived there, too. I shivered, and tossed the
rest of the beets in the garbage. Found a broom and cleaned
up. We wouldn't have beets for Christmas dinner after all.
If my sister-in-law saw this, she would not eat at my table. I
needed her at my table that day.

This would be a Boxing Day project.

I didn't want to tell the boys in the event it slipped out.
Rats could not infest the holiday. Again, this had to be kept
to just me; strange how loneliness had become a presence
in and of itself. My companion. This was not a Christmas
Day thought.

75.

Dinner Pause

We gather at the table
and eat together
no one chokes
we are all alive. Today
is a good day

Around the table
we eat together

Thank you

76

Scratching

CHRISTMAS NIGHT LATE, for the first time, I heard scratching in the walls of the studio as I was trying to fall asleep. The rats were angry, I imagined. So was I. And scared. How should I deal with this? I heard a noise next door in the storeroom. Not for the first time, I longed for my real bedroom, upstairs. But there would still be the rats.

On Boxing Day I cleaned out the storeroom, cleared away any food, re-stacked firewood, made sure the floor was empty, that there were no corners where a rodent would feel safe. Strange how I found a physical metaphor for my mind in this storeroom space, and in the sorting of it. I had mental rats to drive out of my mind. How dare these rodents invade my space. I would create a place of such discomfort. *Fuck you*, came to mind. *You fucking rats.* I was scaring myself with my anger towards the invaders; I could do something to them with my bare hands. Though at the end of the day, there was a certain satisfaction in the arrangements, both in house and mind.

The first day the hardware store was open post-holidays, I was there. I'd watched a ten-minute YouTube video in which a man who bought a condemned house rat-proofed it, made it a home. I wanted to be this man. I bought traps, and steel wool—rats eat it, apparently, and it scrapes out their guts. I didn't care about rat guts. I didn't care how much it hurt them. I bought strong mesh wire to fill any gaps they might have found to come into our home. I bought spray foam that would expand and fill holes. I was armed. Dangerous. I liked it.

I went home, and took a magnifying mirror around the sides of the house, scrutinizing the meeting of siding and concrete foundation. Outside the studio wall there were three rat-sized doorways.

I hoped they were out doing the daytime things rats should be doing on a cold winter's day. I sprayed the foam, and realized the satisfaction of seeing it puff and fill those doorways.

All I had time for that day.

That night, just about to fall asleep, or hoping to at least (Marty was passed out, ear buds in place, podcast whining) and I heard scratching. No! They couldn't be wanting out, they couldn't be trapped in the walls. I held my breath, listening. Then, after some time, the sounds stopped. I realized they were on the outside trying to get in.

Over the next week I used times when people were visiting, or when Marty was watching television with the boys, or napping. I set traps. I removed garden debris from foundation walls. I cleaned and cleared and left everything exposed. I cut branches from eavestroughs. There were no rat-roadways to our house.

On the weekend, my oldest son reported: "There's a mouse in the trap on the roof outside Emmett's room." It's not a mouse, I wanted to say.

There it was, one rat, stiff, dead, pissed off. But its pissed-off-ed-ness—still there in spite of the dead factor—was no match for mine. I left it for others to see, a hanged convict on the walls of the port. *Here you go, Pie-rats!*

Such victory. I had control. I'd won.

One battle, at least.

77.

Boxing Day

is the first time
Marty needs help
in the shower. So
many corners taken
I swear I'm going
in circles

a daily time apart, private to this point
becomes more time together
learning, giving

discovering how to shower another
how to shave a face
how to be another's hands

78.

New Year's Day

MARTY WAS PICKED up and driven to the golf club for the New Year's Day tradition he started so many years ago. The "Chunk-n-Chilly" was a tournament of hungover men that took place every year unless the course was closed for ice and snow. Some years, the guys had to play with brightly coloured balls on a skiff of snow. Mostly, it rained, and the fun was about the complicated rain gear, umbrellas, and full and warming flasks hidden in pockets.

We bundled Marty in blankets and clothing, as light as we could find. Off he went. Happy. Sad and happy. Ole went with him, glad to be of legal age—though that wouldn't have stopped him—and part of the golf club.

I couldn't quite relax into the puttering about the house, though I would have liked to. I listened to music while cleaning up, and made myself dance. A little Earth, Wind & Fire always helps move. I simmered the combination of apples, prunes, raisins on the stove—the "constipation stew" I created to go with Marty's breakfasts. If nothing else, it made the house smell good.

At night, it was late, and I was drifting off to sleep, knowing that the man beside me had had a good day, too. I was suddenly aware of one of those infrequent waves of feeling settled—the day had been a good one. I was relieved to feel this. I had other types of waves, of exhaustion, and of grief. So to know that this type of wave could come, was good. I reminded myself that I would feel this wave again. At some point. The holidays had worn me down in many ways. But had been good in others. In moments.

Out in the rest of the house, I could hear Emmett's voice singing—our in-house Sinatra.

79

Taking it Down

BY THE TIME it was the day to take down the Christmas tree, we were at a point at which I was afraid to touch Marty as he passed by me. In the past I would have reached out with some gesture of affection. He was so unstable now, I hesitated. Also, there was some other shift, under that surface of breathing, but I wasn't sure what it was. Some invisible wall. Something less us. Maybe just that coin with its two sides.

I took down the tree alone, but that wasn't a first. And realized the boys had put only about one quarter of the decorations on it, all the favourite and most delicate glass ones, those I never put on when they were toddlers, or kept above their reach for a tree that glittered waist up. I put them away into the boxes, and fought my mind, trying to envision next Christmas. Which I shouldn't have. But where would we all be?

What will become of me? Marty's words echoed.

The tree was so brittle. A wake of needles followed me out the front door as I tossed it into the rain. I had to struggle to remove the red plastic piece that screwed into the trunk of the tree to set it correctly in the holder. But not as hard as I'd struggled to put it in. I recalled the scene, embarrassed by the mess I was then, and the cursing the neighbours might have heard. I remembered throwing tools around. Now the thing unscrewed so easily. What was the problem those weeks before?

Always, each year, there was the moment of returning into the house, and seeing the empty spot where the tree had been. Some years, I felt a pang, and some a rush of excitement about the new year, and the fillable quality of it. But this year, I paused, looked at the emptiness, felt something well up into me, sad and hard, and I thought, What the fuck kind of Christmas was *that*?!

I thought about the year looming, 2016.

2-0-1-6. All I saw was a date on an obituary. I couldn't see the day or the month, but I could see the year.

Gently, I put my grandmother's star into its 1950s red and green cut-out box, and wondered about the years it had seen. Had it seen any of my grandmother's tears? She had some: a philandering spouse, a stillborn child, a dying toddler. Probably others—many—less obvious and dramatic.

Later, brushing yet more tree needles off the window seat—they were everywhere—I found the long shoehorn I'd bought for Marty in the summer. I remembered my euphoria—no less—with finding it back then. It seemed to answer the issue at that moment; but that moment shifted. As did the issue. Tectonic plates.

In the middle of the night, the day after New Year's Day, I awoke, and my mind began to churn. How we wasted so many years taking each other for granted. Often when my thoughts turned in that direction, I could move myself to the last while—before Marty got sick—the time in which I thought we'd made up for the years that came before. I cried. My tears woke up Marty, and he cried too.

Happy New Year.

My phone burbled, and I saw a text from a friend that said the same.

80.

2016

TOWARD THE END of the holidays, Ole decided that home was the place he needed to be, and he let his golf coach know (he was on athletic scholarship) and signed up for online classes through his university. Although he didn't want to say so at first, Marty admitted that he was happy Ole had made this decision.

Cleve visited us every weekend, after his long Monday-to-Friday hours, and Emmett was the best sixteen-year-old nurse ever. And now it was good to have Ole back home with us. He called the walker "Dad's whip" and made him laugh. He made sound effects—wheels turning sharply and skidding—as his dad trundled by and made all of us laugh.

Each boy had a role, different, and significant. At times I recalled that when I was unexpectedly pregnant for the third time, I wondered at how I could possibly love three children as much as I loved two. What parts would I have to tear from what was in place for the two to make room. Then I experienced the elasticity of love. I needed to see and feel anew that elasticity now. Caregiving demanded elasticity.

As we set out into the new year of 2016, I questioned how it was the sadness that was overwhelming. Anger or a sense of unfairness would be easier to live with. But sadness would keep me human, while anger and bitterness would make me miserable. The sadness deep in my husband was harder to accept, though; his loss was so much greater than mine.

81.

January Punctuation

Marty gets up this morning to use the loo
and as he pushes his walker across the floor
he lets out a stream of squeaky farts
They come to an end just
as he reaches the door, and just
as I let go one
—an exclamation mark to end his sentence
"So there!" I say, and he laughs

82

Team 7

I AWOKE ONE night, wide awake from a dream or thought. This was around the time that Marty's speech was becoming increasingly difficult to understand. He could still text and write on his iPad, but messages were growing shorter for the effort they required. The dream—or the thought I was left with, at least—was that I couldn't remember how one of my two older boys said the phrase "belly button." Really, I couldn't even remember that this had been some particular phrase. That wasn't the point; the point was the panic on wakening, the panic at being left as the sole repository of memories. Marty had been the family archivist, the photographer, the videographer. I'd scribbled notes here and there, but had often found myself—regrettably, as a writer—short on time for a daily journal.

What other memories was I losing? Who would sit with me and reminisce? In my life, where would go the phrase "Remember when..."? Back in the summer, by the fire, we'd shared an evening of reminiscing about Ole's imaginary friend (named—imaginatively—Chris), and about how Emmett didn't speak until almost three years of age. I'd reminded Marty about Jesus, Emmett's pet snail, who would wander out of his bowl of water and cedar frond, make his way around the living room on adventures, and always return to life once returned to his bowl; once he even went missing under the couch for several months, and dried to being weightless. I discovered him after vacuuming (I don't vacuum under couches too often). Emmett chanced upon this, even as I was thinking to toss before being discovered, and demanded that Jesus be returned to the bowl. Which I did. Wondering how long it might take to go outside and find a Jesus substitute, a lively one.

Ten minutes later, Jesus was trolling the edges of the bowl, antennae up and happy as shit. Returned from the dead.

83.

Lean In

I lean in for a kiss
at the close of the day, after
tucking him into bed

When I pull away
the expression in his eyes is odd
"Do you need a hug?" I ask, and he says
a hug makes it hard to breathe. No

Takes me a minute to understand the words, longer to
absorb, especially
the last one. I leave the room to cry

84.

Bright Bits

WAS IT BEING not even a couple of weeks into a new year that had me pondering what matters most? What mattered to me?

Whether Marty had peaceful sleep.

Whether Ole had a good evening with a teammate—something that brought him back home with a lightness in his step.

Whether Emmett still sang as he went about the house.

Whether our dinner tasted as it should—pizza, home-made in January for the first time in too long; I swore it only tasted as it should with thought put into it, in addition to the more obvious ingredients.

Even that small piece mattered. I'd had this discussion several times with my husband over the years: how pizza, and so much food, tasted better if I took time with it. It was slowing, and preparing it with thought and care that infused food with flavour. We'd disagreed on this. But he'd always been happy to eat my Saturday night pizza.

Maybe I did go too far when I said that dogs were capable of looking embarrassed or pleased or the myriad of canine expressions possible. I still believed that, but Marty would chuckle and say it was all in my head.

Pizza and dogs aside... What mattered?

Had I been kind to people? Now there was a big one. I was struggling with this. Maybe it was the biggest. Would Marty's last thoughts be filled with family and love and warmth? The things that would build this *were* small, I suspected—making tea at the right moment, taking time to dress him so nothing hurt, combing his hair so we could laugh over some resemblance to Steve Buscemi. But I was conscious of building to that last moment. I pushed back at the possibility that such actions didn't matter. They had to. It was unbearable to think they might not.

I have a poignant memory of being age seven, with my head on my mother's lap, looking through the windshield—of what, the Dodge dart or the VW van that came next?—and seeing stars. Seatbelts were no concern then; stars mattered.

The sky behind the stars was that deepest blue-black, with no clouds, or not in my memory. Just layers of endless bright bits. They were beautiful. After all my parents' talk of heaven, I looked out at the bank of stars, and a feeling spread through me. I remember that mostly: inside me, and around me, contentment.

Now, this was being tested.

When I further mined the memory, I recalled how at that age I was not only questioning in my gut, but I'd begun to try to articulate. "Mom, if God created the world, where did God come from?" I remember her flapping panic more than I remember her exact words. She wanted that question to go away. Toothpaste back in tube. I had a lot of questions:

"What do you mean when you say God and Jesus are *inside* us?" My mother told me about heaven, about hell, about living forever to praise God after we die. I didn't remember being brave enough to ask the same questions of my father.

A few years before I turned seven, my father had given up on the church we'd attended, the church in which he and my mom had met and married, and he opted for his own Sunday school at home, to which we invited neighbour kids. He would then read Bible chapters, and we progressed through as the months and years passed. My mother ordered hymnals, one for each of us. Or were there more? Did we just share with visitors? I don't remember. I don't remember there being any questions about any of this.

I remember my father unhappy that I couldn't—he thought "wouldn't"—sing loud enough to be heard. He demanded I sing. I was so upset that I left the room in tears, and crawled under my bed, a four-poster affair with substantial space beneath it. I looked out to see his shoes and trouser hems after he followed me, and I could hear his voice, frustrated, telling me to come out, to come back to the living room, and to sing louder because he knew I could. Which did not inspire any urge to reappear and rejoin, if that's what he intended.

The memory is strongly etched into my mind, as a moment of significant doubt about this religion stuff. Why be angry with someone for not singing loudly enough? What was important? How could this matter?

That night, when I was seven and looking at the stars through the windshield, it came to me that they were only stars out there. There wasn't heaven hiding behind them. There wasn't backstage. Just stars forever, reaching back and out and all around. Hundreds, thousands, maybe more. Hard to think of such numbers as a kid more drawn to words. But maybe this was the eternal I'd been hearing about. Shiny little bright bits in the sky. Maybe they were heaven.

Why did there need to be more? I still thought that. Or at least, I'd thought I did—that if I looked at them, if I matched my breathing with theirs, they were enough. But the awareness of the matching, the breathing—where did that come from?

If I could wheel Marty out in that chair to look up and see them, what would he feel? Would he feel the "enough"? What was it that had given me the sense of contentment? What was the missing piece? Was there a missing piece? It was as if we'd made a puzzle, something complicated, and found, at the end, that we were missing one piece.

Neither Mary nor Martha seemed capable of a half answer.

85.

Cold Day in January

THIS DAY CAME, and I went into the ALS Clinic on my own. The one time I did.

I went to spend a couple of hours being instructed on dealing with a feeding tube. The success of the feeding tube, and staying at home—the ultimate carrot—was dependent on my learning to use it. I'd had no idea what a PEG tube was. Percutaneous endoscopic gastrostomy. A soft, flexible tube that takes food stuff into the gut. It is inserted through an opening in the abdomen, and the tube goes directly into the stomach. It works well to feed and medicate while bypassing mouth and esophagus. The surgery involved would take mere minutes, and then we were to spend the night in the hospital for observation, and to make certain I could manage the use and cleaning of the tube.

I was one of those mothers who never did master the art of a thermometer in the mouth and reading it. I was more apt to look at a paled child and measure listlessness as indicative of fever, than to work with a bit of glass and mercury. Glass and mercury scared me. Feeding tube paraphernalia looked daunting. Impossible, really.

I remember that training day clearly, the ease of it. I remember walking out of my house, stopping to look up at the bare wintry trees. Every time I was outside, I paused, let the sky, the air, the trees, the smell of soil, soak in to me. I couldn't not do that in those months. I'd soak enough so it could stay with me, or try to at least, until the next time I was on the outer side of the front door.

It was so quick to get into my car, with just me. I could drive slowly, unassertively. Or however I wanted. Yet that didn't feel necessarily good; just felt what it was.

Then it struck me, once I pulled into the parking lot at GF Strong: I didn't have to find the nearest space. In fact, I'd best leave the nearest for someone who needed it. So I parked in the farthest, and enjoyed the walk. Felt a twinge of guilt in enjoying the walk. But was also aware of how, like looking to the sky, and absorbing the brief times in the outdoor air, I needed such sustaining moments. They weren't a luxury. It seemed only seconds passed and I was in the elevator to the basement. Always so keenly aware of those wheeling about in chairs. Their ages. Young people. I appreciated efforts that I saw in these people to dress with imagination. In the last few years of my life before this major turn, I'd learned the importance of seeing one's body as a canvas for colour, and as a fine place to show one's own. Splash.

I moved easily through the clinic door, announced I was there. No pushing chair, no straightening or removal of the winter poncho. There was no other person to pay attention to. It was the oddest feeling. I felt it, and simultaneously was aware of this at every moment, as if a ghost person was next to me.

Before we got to the training with the dietician, the nurse talked with me. I can't remember how we got to the conversation. I only remember that we were talking about something else, possibly something quite innocuous. Perhaps the new year; it was still only January. Holiday talk was still possible. But suddenly she was telling me about what it would be like: *The End*. Big music swell.

Did she plan this talk? Did she know how to start in one place in conversation, and end up in another? Or was it more instinct... and she knew I was ready? At one point she asked if I'd like for her to stop. Or go on. Please go on, I said. I need to know this. Yet a moment before it hadn't occurred to me that she would tell me, and that I needed to know right now how it would be. (Always a sense of movement, of push. Of grabbing at what came up, because I had to trust it was coming up for a reason, and I needed to pay attention to both the thing at hand and the reason.)

Somewhere in my mind I could hear Dr. K's words about this being the poster disease for physician-assisted death, dying with dignity, assisted suicide—all the terms—and how everything about ALS would be exaggerated. I recalled his words about ignoring the television portrayal of this disease, the media stuff.

I listened to the nurse now, and she was echoing Dr. K. "It's peaceful," she said. "Usually in sleep."

That caused a sense of new panic in me. Really? He'd die in his sleep? I'd awake to find him gone? I couldn't possibly go through all this to find him gone, slipped away, without me knowing. Hearing this, on my own, was strange. I was already in a strange headspace that day, with being on my own. "On my own" felt heightened somehow with her words. I could feel the space beside me grow. That's what this was about for me, that's where it was going. To be *on my own.*

In the meantime, there was this business of the feeding tube, the administering of it. I was always holding on to at least two pieces. Juggling. (Dodging? Only when I dropped?)

But I listened as she explained how morphine works, the double edges of it, so sharp you can't feel it cutting: the capacity to lessen breathing, the capacity to lessen anxiety about the lessened breathing. Lessening. Word of the day, brought to you by the letter L.

I was glad someone finally took time to explain to me what Marty's last moments might look like. That the gasping and choking I'd imagined was not the right picture to hold. That there was palliative medication that did what it prom-ised to. I've never had much faith in medication, and there was so little that ameliorated anything about this disease. But this part of it sounded tested and true. Pain would not be an issue. At least, not physical pain. There was something of value in all this, and I held on to it.

"Carbon dioxide accumulates," she went on, "and makes the person sleepy. At some point they simply don't have enough oxygen, or even want it, and they fall asleep." She paused. "Some people's partners have described it as a 'rest-ful death'." Her words settled into me.

I really had not realized the relief that would come with this knowledge. Well-timed and delivered knowledge is a gift. I took it as such. It even made the feeding tube seem easier. Oddly.

I'd believed there was no dignity with this disease— although it is an admirable thing to try to hold on to it in spite of that knowledge. In *that* lies the dignity. It was necessary to hold on to the belief in the possibility that one could create as much dignity as possible.

The nurse left, the dietician came in, and we began our lesson. I became a note-taking student, a role I was used to. I took visual footage of the steps too, with my phone. I practiced. I held the pieces—the tubing, the plastic bags that I looped over the twisty hooks on the IV pole. Was this me doing this?

At one point in the lesson I heard myself saying "right" and "okay"—offering affirmatives to indicate that I understood, that I could do this. Suddenly I had an urge just to wail. Just to sit in the middle of that floor, in that godforsaken basement, with the shit sunshine-slithering-through-forest-trees mural on the wall, and wail. Who was I in this person who was so practical? Who could think she'd be okay doing this... this tube thing? Giving these medications? And being all Cherry Ames, the mystery novel nurse-heroine I'd grown up with? Who was this Cherry Ames-me? Did I know her? What was the difference between someone who nodded and said "right" and someone who would fall to pieces? Why was I one and not the other? What hairline of difference was there? Was the hairline always in me, or had I built it somehow? When? How? Why? I felt short of breath, as if my lungs had been taken hold of, some nasty hands squeezing them small, and me trying to push air into them. (Was this what *his* lungs felt? Such thoughts came to my mind throughout the days, always seeking to understand, and unable to know.)

Still I said right and okay, and yes, strangely I understood. I knew that, armed with my little phone videos of instruction, I would be what I needed to be. I would be Martha, wide-hipped and able. Hand-tossed pizza dough over my shoulder. Ready to march.

Sometimes Martha hovered over me as I hand-wrote in my journal. I got the feeling she was fussing over something. Sometimes, in the deep hours, I swore I heard her typing. She couldn't sit and just do nothing. Couldn't daydream. No, she was always *doing*.

Just sit. Be still.

But perhaps her being was all in her doing.

86.

Communications Folks

WHAT DO COMMUNICATIONS experts do when they come to visit, bringing yet another iPad of Official, Expensive, and Appropriate Software on it for eased communication with Marty?

They yell.

I almost laughed aloud. But restrained myself. Everything the woman said was at louder-than-necessary volume. I wanted to say, "Marty is not deaf!" but kept my peace. I also would have liked to remind them (team of two) that ALS can be akin to living in a concussed state which cannot stand over-stimulation. So if people are shouting or moving too fast it just hurts.

On that first visit they brought over an enormous stand (a tubular affair big enough to go around the base of the Archie Bunker recliner) intended to hold the iPad to the right of the arm rest, only to assemble it and realize it was missing the tiny piece intended to hold the iPad in place. Rather than take it apart, they set it to one side of the living room, and then left the house with the promise to "requisition" the missing piece.

I knew it would never happen. As an academic in an institution, the word "requisition" never bodes well in my experience. A colleague once borrowed a 79-cent rubber door stopper from a nearby department to save us the grief of requisitioning one for our own department; it was fair, we thought, to give Philosophy something to ponder.

I went into Marty's collection of musical equipment, found the sturdiest music stand we had, and set it up to hold the iPad; it fulfilled the task quite adequately, took little space, and made sense. Later, it even multi-tasked, and took on the job of holding the bag of urine, too. No requisitioning required.

Martha gave a smart nod on this.

87

Rosebud

I LOOKED UP at the "Rosebud" sled, high on the wall of our living room, over the fireplace. With cabin-like, cedar interior, we had the sled, as well as snowshoes. My dad had fastened the sled there after my mother found it, discarded by a neighbour, and hauled it home with love. (Or maybe with regret, since she'd thrown out an identical one, on which we tore down the hills in the sixties and early seventies.)

That sled was from a time of innocence. Not just from the time we used one as children, but even when we fastened it to the wall. For holidays, I'd attached lights to it, or boughs from red twig dogwood bushes, or large glass-like snowflakes. But now I looked at it, and it mocked me in some way. Or did it sorrow with me? I reminded myself to be gentle with me. It was too easy to imagine one way, possible mocking, when in fact it could well be another. Go gently when life is pushing you.

Those old sleds were tough to steer. In those days, there was a track to the side of the slope, on which sledders trudged up to the top, keeping well away from those heading breakneck down. Back then we were smart enough to know to keep out of their way. Once started, there was little predicting their paths. They'd just go. The only way to do otherwise—other than down at top speed—was to bail out, tuck in your head, and hope the snow didn't go too far down the neck of your jacket, or that you didn't blow a boot.

I lived in my house and saw things in ways I'd never seen before. Something could be from one time, and now felt to be part of another. Things—simple things—began to disconnect. It was unnerving. Disequilibrium. They say that's the state for learning.

88.

Timing

TIMING WAS EVERYTHING, and I sought a moment to share with Marty "the end" as described by the nurse at the clinic. Maybe another of his "What will become of me?" questions would come as an entry-point. Instead, while talking over plans for the one hospital stay—the installation of the feeding-tube—it seemed a fit. A moment at the breakfast table, while eating, and conversation had turned to the purported ease that he looked forward to with the advent of the tube. I shared what the nurse had told me. I spoke bluntly, and didn't repeat myself. It took only seconds, but I could see the relief in him. He'd been envisioning the same nasty goodbye that I had been. I wished I could have told him earlier, and not tiptoed looking for the chink in his wall. But if I'd told him at another moment, one not so right, he might have grown angry with the reminder that there was going to be an end, or with the fact that I'd held on to the information for some days.

It can be hard to read the face with ALS. On every level, my ability to read him was deteriorating, too. When some piece of timing worked, I was grateful.

89

After Monday, There's Tuesday

SOMEONE WITH A kind heart loaned me *Tuesdays With Morrie*, and I read about an ageing man, academic and pontificating. So many words. The sheer number of words spoken by the man in that book indicated a different ALS experience from the one we were in the midst of. I did appreciate his words about spending moments each morning with a jag of grieving his self—acknowledging—before going on with his day. That was a peace-offering of wisdom.

In January, friends brought over a novel, something they'd just read and enjoyed, *All the Light We Cannot See*. It was as if I were a child again, suddenly, with that read, back when reading was not a part of my job, when reading was getaway joy.

It was still that, in the midst of never leaving the house except to pick up meds and bananas and milk. People brought over everything else.

Another friend, from several provinces away, mailed me a book he'd just finished reading, and it too was joy, sad book though it was. (Unknown to me at that time was that this particular friend had just been diagnosed with a recurrence of cancer and had decided to keep the knowledge close; I had no idea. He passed away not many months after Marty.)

The book was *Fifteen Dogs* by André Alexis. It meant something that these books had been previously read by the givers, and were then handed to me with thought.

Remembering what reading could be for me became one of the gifts of this time.

90

Kleenex

When did Kleenex become part
of our lives? I made it through
having three boys. Never
had one in a pocket or my purse; I used to joke
I wasn't a real mother
If a boy had a nose to blow, use TP
I've bought a box now and then of extra soft ones
if someone has a rattling, snorting cold, but otherwise
just never made it to the grocery list
Now tissues are everywhere
Kitchen table. By the TV. The counter. Desks
Like an old peoples' home, is how I see it
To catch tears and honk noses
I remember to put one in my pocket
before a walk
I load up at the drugstore, say
to the young woman cashiering
"I hate needing these"
She laughs as if I've said
something funny

91.

Picnic

ON JANUARY 14, we drove to UBC Hospital, found the gastro-enterology unit, bottom floor. There was all the business of getting into a hospital gown, clothing folded away, shoes off, wrist band on. I was suddenly aware of what it might be like to have a partner with a different type of illness; I'd not thought of this to date. There were illnesses with different steps to them, some small, some large, some that might bring points of healing or some sort of repair, and with them, possibly, some hope. What was that like? When you took a step and it brought a positive result? What was it to live with that? When you might return from a hospital stay feeling you'd accomplished something? I pulled the thought through my mind, an imagined glimpse of others' lives.

What were *we* doing here, though, with the PEG tube thing? A delay tactic, for the most part. I had a lingering feeling that this was not the right step. Of wishing the specialist had spelled out in detail the results of both scenarios: the one he had shared, "life with tube," and also the one he did not share or illustrate: "life without tube." When he shared what it would be like, describing how the tube would enter Marty's abdomen, what it would look like, how it would work, Marty had quickly said, "Let's do it!" with all the enthusiasm of purchasing a concert ticket. I'd wished the specialist would spell out what this choice would mean—that life would be extended, but could he draw another picture of what that would *be*?

I could have articulated the picture with the research I'd done. But I was the spouse; I didn't want to have to be the picture-drawer, too. Even if I drew the picture, would Marty see it? Or I could draw, but didn't want to have to explain. It shouldn't have to be my job to do this. It should have been the specialist's. How could there be informed choice with only one picture? I had the feeling, at that moment in the specialist's office, that if I did indeed articulate Option 2, I would also have to explain, interpret, and that would make me the Bad Guy. Did I misjudge? There were so many times I had to be Bad Guy that I was reluctant to blunder into yet another. The task of judging my husband's cognitive capacity was a challenge. He was not so impaired that he couldn't feel manipulated, and then resentment. When he embraced something, showed enthusiasm, I stepped back.

Sometimes I thought about Dr. K's words, about starvation not being a terrible death. He'd said this when the discussion of "tube" first came up in late fall. But his words were either unheard by Marty, or he'd chosen to ignore.

So. There we were.

Let's go back to the night before.

When I was tucking him into bed, he said, "I'm scared."

"I'm scared, too," I said. My mind worked through what it needed to, returning to a passage in a book I'd read, about how to drill down to the nature of fear, rather than simply accepting. About how to narrow the defining of fear, as opposed to some general scary shit thing that would seem too big to live with.

"What are you afraid of?" I asked. The question stopped my own tears.

"Pain," he said.

That was still too big.

But I'd learned not to open possibilities with my questions. I attempted to clarify, beginning with the most innocuous: "Do you mean the pain of the tube being installed?" (Even as I heard the echo in my own head, about the Other Thing, the pain of leaving this life.)

"Yes," was the answer. So it was the immediate, the simpler. The do-able.

I repeated what both the specialist and the dietician at the Clinic had said, about how painkillers would be administered in a timely manner. The pain would be minimal, I reassured. I would be watching the time and the amounts, I promised. It would be about setting a timer on my phone, about watching him for signs of further exhaustion. (If only I'd thought to slip a bottle of Tylenol into my purse. *Be careful what you promise.*)

But the night before, falling asleep, asserting an answer to his anxiety about pain, he looked at peace about the immediate future. I couldn't ask for more. I set an alarm to awake in an hour and forty minutes, at 11:00 PM, so he could have a last bite of food before Cut Off time for fasting prior to the procedure. Crisis and tears averted for the moment.

THE ALARM WENT off, and Marty was as much asleep as I had been awake for the hour and some.

In the kitchen, I prepared slices of banana on a red plate, each with a small dollop of peanut butter. Comfort food. On the kitchen table, Emmett was happily gaming, and I was thankful for his presence. Just before I returned to the studio-bedroom, I grabbed a lantern candleholder; the overhead light was too harsh to break Marty's sleep. He'd need more solid sleep before the morning.

In the room, I set the candle on the bedside shelf, and tried to awaken him, feeling pangs of having to break what was, for once, a deep sleep. He finally awakened, and I hugged him gently, loosely, as I pulled him into a seated position. I put my short black robe around his shoulders as it was lighter than the long red one I'd bought for him recently, and I pulled his cardigan over his knees. I sat on the edge of the bed beside him. The lantern had star-shaped cut-outs in its surface, and these cast kindly and flickering shadows on the ceiling and walls, and I was struck by how oddly right it felt to have a midnight picnic, aside from the intentions of this particular one. Why was it that I'd never woken him up before for such a thing? Why didn't people just do this once in a while? How was it this had never occurred to me? The thought was an unexpected gift, with a bit of dreamer Mary in it.

I fed him the rounds of banana. He had sips of water. He was hungry and ate too quickly. Several times I asked him to slow down—he was making me nervous.

He finished and said something with an S sound. Might have been the word "nice." I asked him to repeat, and hated how I had to ask him again and again to repeat words. "Great snack."

In the morning, he spooned around me. Would this be possible with a tube protruding from his gut? (It was; the tube was soft. It was the breathing that got in the way.)

Pluses of the tube: no more choking, or struggling to breathe at mealtimes. Not having to eat, to lift a utensil, which had come to feel like a weight, then to chew and swallow. All this meant his energy wouldn't be utterly depleted after even just a snack. This was good, I told myself. I told myself a lot of things.

But another thought came on the heels of this, in the way that thoughts do flit from one subject to another, with only the most tenuous thread connecting: this, that we were now past the point of ever being able to have an in-depth conversation. True, it had been that way for some weeks now, but thoughts take time to catch up. Which was just as well. I could only handle so many thoughts at a time. At times, many times, I'd like to turn off my mind altogether. I focused on the mental images I played through my mind, reminding myself who he was, the images that kept me human. Midnight picnics would keep us human.

IN THE MIDDLE of the night, the one night hospital stay, the nurse did not show up with the painkillers I'd promised Marty. One regular strength Tylenol could not be produced in a timely manner. The nurse, new on her shift, was busy reading over the records. "I need to be certain he hasn't had too many pills," she said. "Liver damage, you know," she whispered, conspiratorially. I stood in front of her, in my midnight stocking feet, and looked her in the eye. "He has ALS," I said. "So liver damage isn't the issue."

"Oh," was all she said. Almost forty minutes passed before she tripped down the hall to bring the medication. Perhaps she was a slow reader. Which seemed out of synch with the rest of the hospital stay experience, much of which seemed a whirlwind.

The abrupt movement of the nurses left an impression on me. Were they aware of it? It spoke of a lack of patience and care—though in reality, it probably had more to do with getting on with the mass of tasks before them. One did manage to move quickly, and yet maintain a calming nature; did she consciously work at that? It was admirable. But more often than not, their speech cut off Marty's and my own, as they completed our staggered sentences. I hadn't realized how we had slowed. This was a revelation. For decades I'd lived with Marty's fast pace. An evening out for him meant stopping in at several clubs to see friends performing, or checking out more than one party to wish someone happy birthday. An evening in one place was a rarity. Now we were like two old tumbleweeds, drifted into a fence and caught, while others swirled round.

Earlier, preparing for the night, another nurse was showing us her favourite way to turn a patient in bed. Each nurse on the ward appeared to have a unique way to do this, and each, as a result, felt exorbitantly superior to the other nurses, in spite of being work-mates. At one point during her show, Marty barked at me, some order I couldn't make out. He yelled again. He was in pain with the abdominal incision, I reminded myself. Even I was irritated by my lack of ability to understand his speech. The nurse's head snapped up, and she stared at him. She said something about being emphatic, and he said he had to be; that much was clear. I was embarrassed, hurt, even as part of me struggled to find where he was, in his pain, in his cognitive mush. I wished, rather irrationally, that the nurse had had a bit more crone in her, and could snap back at him, say something about being nice to his wife. But where was my spine, I wondered, that I resisted doing that for myself? How did one stand up to a dying person, a dying person in pain? Or do you stand up?

THE NEXT DAY, Dr. K visited. He greeted us, then left the room for a moment to talk with someone. While he was out, Marty said, "Tell Doc I want to die." He repeated himself, but for once I'd heard the words the first time. I did have to ask him to repeat himself as he spoke further, though, and agitation set in. "I can't talk!" He motioned to the doorway. "Go tell him!"

I was shaking when I went to meet Dr. K in the hallway, and repeated. The doctor looked thoughtful. "Everyone wants to die in the hospital," he said. It was not yet time, he added. How would we know when it *was* time? Marty's speech was going so quickly. We'd signed the paperwork that gave me certain rights, along with power of attorney. But how would I *know*? I could not decide such a thing. I'd always voiced glib words about what I would do if, but here I was. The thought of the reality, of making that decision for another, didn't seem real or possible.

ONCE HOME FROM the hospital, there was a shift in Marty's abilities, and I began to have to help him up and down on chairs and the toilet, and to get his water bottle for him at night. Through January, his speech worsened. He uttered less and less. As a result, the house was quieted, movement slowed. The sense of stillness and silence grew. At times I had the sensation of floating through the rooms, through my life even. But that was not a long period in time; nature abhors a vacuum.

It became the thing to do, for Marty to creep up the volume on the television or radio, until those sounds filled the house and the rafters. Until, not many weeks of this later, I thought I'd go mad with the sound. After their dad passed away, if our sons were sitting watching something together, one of them would say, "Here's Dad!" and bring the television volume to a full 46. They'd share this memory, and a warm laugh, and then turn it back down. Legacy.

92.

Life With Tube

THE FEEDING TUBE brought with it a new time of procedure. Rinsing and cleaning the bags and storing them in the fridge between feedings. At first, we didn't use the tube for feeding. The specialist and Dr. K said it was ideal to put the tube in before it was really necessary for eating, so that it would be in place for both food and medication when needed, and while his body still had strength to heal, and he was able to get around the hospital. That meant daily flushing and care of the tube in the meantime.

The apparatus of IV pole on wheels, together with the onslaught of hospital furnishings, in the midst of living room, was all so strange. One day, looking for something upstairs, I came across the furry dice Cleve had left behind when he moved out, and after selling me his car, and when I picked them up, ready to toss, a thought came to me, and I took them downstairs and hung them on the IV pole. "Your new wheels," I said to Marty, and got a weak smile out of him. My goal at that point was to get at least one of those each day. You had to know how such a smile appears to recognize it; the slightest pull at the corners of his mouth.

Possibly just in his eyes, and that was how we translated it, his boys and I. My mind was getting used to looking for objects, details, quick stories, to make this smile come. To achieve some light in those eyes.

Dr. K laughed, too, when he saw those furry dice. So did the boys.

93.

Together

Cleve and Emmett
put together the towel rack I ordered
for the new bathroom, plans and pieces
set out over the living room floor. Today
Emmett helps Ole sort through his online computer
course. Tonight
Cleve is taking his brothers to see *Star Wars* in the
theatre
Our boys are so different
from each other. And they are
working together
I marvel at this

94.

Blue

IT WAS ANOTHER Monday, and I had the becoming-too-familiar feeling of being brittle. I had many days with this feeling. To a lesser degree I'd felt this way some years before, when I was stretched at work, so many needs with children, and overwhelmed. But this had added layers: the constant levels of need, all of almost equal tending, and sorting out that "almost"—what should be done now, what could be put off. Dealing with the new layer of feeding tube, reading directions, realizing I hadn't interpreted—could I even understand simple written directions? How to interpret the appearance of... whatever it was... in the tube. Always dealing with a type of anxiety that lay low for the most part, but was a constant: Was I doing what I should be, and was I doing it correctly?

How to describe the brittleness. As if the lightest wind could blow, and I'd come to pieces; a constant sense of holding it together. Just barely.

The ALS Clinic folks had suggested neck collars for support, and we had two different sizes in the house. That day, with Marty working at his desk, I put one on at his request.

Worked to adjust it. Asked him how it felt. He barked at me (granted, everything came out as a bark—it was his new voice. But this really was a bark that would have been a bark, regardless) that he didn't know yet, he'd barely worn it.

He was quite right in this; the thing had been on for minutes only. But it hurt, the tone and the words. The impatience. I left the room.

I helped Ole with some studying for an exam. I called the occupational therapist about equipment needs: what we needed and what we needed to get rid of. Took a student's thesis to the post office while Marty was napping. I did the daily rat trap check on the roof. And cleaned the kitchen.

Later, I realized Marty had typed an "I'm sorry" text to me. It helped, but there was still an ache that didn't go away.

On the radio at dinnertime, I heard that it was Blue Monday, the most depressing day of the year.

So.

I wasn't so out of touch with the outside world after all.

95.

Shower Chair

THE ALS SOCIETY folks brought us a large—very large—wheeled commode-and-shower chair.

Its sheer size made me gulp. It was white and grey plastic, with red plastic brakes on all four wheels, and a cutout in the bottom of the seat, with grey commode pot under. It looked like some strange robotic thing without a head. No, it had a headrest. Robot without a face.

It looked complicated.

Marty was at the breakfast table, where he'd been since I talked him into forestalling his shower to wait for the arrival of this new chair. But at that moment, I wished we'd done one last morning with the flimsy plastic shower chair we'd been working with since just before Christmas, white and teal, with its thin aluminum legs, useless-looking suction cups on each. It looked ready to come to pieces, and I hadn't wanted to put it to any test.

This new thing was just big. It looked as if it had Stuff to Figure Out. Sometimes—more often now—my brain was just tired of Figuring Out.

(Yet every morning of maneuvering the handrail and the light plastic chair was a time of held breath, hoping nothing happened. *Please don't slip.* So I'd have to be willing to trade Figuring Out for Fear-Filled Breath-Holding.)

To buy time, I gathered Marty's clothing to warm over the heat duct. Last ditch effort: I went upstairs on some pretext. Then slumped against the wall in the hall, and sat on the floor to give myself a moment. Wimp, I thought. On so many counts. Not the least of which: He can't follow me up here. Tears gathered but did not spill. Damn, they would not spill. This robot thing had to be less complicated than the actual wheelchair, I told myself. I'd figured out that; I could figure out this.

I realized though that while all my life I could remember seeing wheelchairs—probably from the first mention of Clara's wheeled chair in my childhood favourite book, *Heidi*—I had no experience whatsoever with its more private cousin, the wheeled shower commode, generally hidden out of sight. Multi-tasking piece of hell.

Back downstairs. Why, looking at it, did I have a sense that it hid secrets? While I was intensely grateful to those ALS Society warehouses everywhere, there was something to the shared quality of the pieces: My mind went to who might have had this before us. And who would have it after. The word "after" stuck. What sorrows were absorbed into the pieces? What stories?

Life had grown to be always about change. True, this is what life is, but at that point it was too obvious; the changes were relentless. What would come after The Shower Chair? I stopped my mind at that. I was getting fairly good at stopping my mind. This was, after all, a crash course in living in the moment. That thing people preach. Or pacing it to move slowly. To slow the mind while one's narrow world marches along, or runs.

I touched a lever—looked as if it might have something to do with tilting it back—and jumped when the entire thing jerked into recline. It took minutes and struggle to find the way back to upright. *If I'd done that with Marty in it...* Stop the mind.

Marty sent me a text to request that I warm up the chair in the steamy water. Right—good suggestion. I did. And forgot to pull out the commode pot, before moving him from the seat on the walker to the shower chair. We went through the shower routine, and then when I pulled the chair out of the shower, into the room, the pot rolled out, with water everywhere.

I grabbed towels and heading-for-laundry-anyway clothing to mop up, and was grateful that we'd tiled the entire room with a splash border all around. Even as the water leaked toward the door.

By the time I was finished, and it felt to be mere minutes, Marty's toes were purple with cold in spite of the warm and dry towels I'd thrown over him before I began the mop up. I'd lifted him back onto the walker seat (we never really used the wheelchair inside the house; the walker seat was enough), and in moving him, I was too quick, and hurt his shoulder. At that point, the muscles in his left shoulder had loosened to the point of almost dislocation. Tears filled his eyes. I took extra long, bending over him, to pull on sweatpants and socks, to hide my own tears. I was so sorry to hurt him, to make such a mess of things. Everything felt to be so rushed, rushing, rushing along. The room was slippery wet and dangerous. He was cold and needed clothing and a light blanket. There was the need for the balance of slow and quick. Warmth was priority. But so was not causing pain. Everything coincided.

Really, I needed to sit and have a cup of slow coffee. Though that wouldn't be for months. I had to find internal ways to slow. Four years of yoga breathing kicked in, and did help. But...

What are the acts and rituals we have throughout our days that result in a consistent strengthening of our selves? Or at least maintenance? My morning coffee. Thinking time. Walking. Simple things that are easy to take for granted.

Through the grieving months after Marty passed, I sought out music as refuge, as light. Old music, new. Jazz, blues. Artists I'd never heard of until then. Music became a constant with me. But when I was in the depths of caregiving, with Marty's preference for the television and radio, with my own discomfort with ear-buds, it never occurred to me to listen. It might have created the mental and emotional space that it did later. To be able to take time to mull over one's needs seemed a luxury. There was no time to consider what would put some energy into the well-spring. The well was running dry, and when it did bring up some water, it was mud, and I was choking on it.

96.

Flamenco Baseline

SHORTLY AFTER I took up yoga, I'd also begun dance classes, and discovered flamenco in my late forties. Its initial appeal for me was its history. It was the dance of the Romani who hid in caves to keep from persecution. Their dances were emotional: the *bulerias,* a party dance, with joy and tease; the *solea,* with sorrow; the *siguiriyas,* with despair. The history reached to me, hauled me in, and in spite of almost five decades of timing issues, I started classes. The idea of creating such noise, stamping, clapping, voices keening in those caves in the cliffs of Andalusia, while hiding from death—that caught me. I never danced as a child, for the same reason we went without television for those years. Dance was Sin, in my growing-up home. Which quite possibly made me enjoy it more as an adult.

Flamenco was the third form of dance that I tried; it was the one that reached my gut and answered questions I didn't know I was asking. The decade of my forties was spent facing professional failure. After years of teaching post-secondary successfully, I could not pass the critical eyes of those who scrutinize candidates for an education degree to teach grade school. My writing career was always butting up against the teaching, and slowly my weight crept up to a point where I noticed it while tying my shoes and on lengthy walks. (Why do some middle-aged women hide behind weight? Some inversion of anorexia?)

Change was slow. My food habits were the first on the examination table, and it took thirty months to lose thirty pounds. They stayed away after that. Yoga, and then dance, became key in this metamorphosis and self-knowledge. The positive turn that my marriage took was no doubt part of this, too, as everything works together. All of this—the failure, the listening to my gut, the care of my physical and emotional self—had prepared me for what was now happening. All the pieces played roles. I noticed this. I was grateful. Five years earlier, I would have been a mess. Or more of a mess.

Even as life cartwheeled, and I scrambled, I still made it to three dance classes each week, hanging on, hanging on. Flamenco had had a healing effect on me, and I knew that I would need it in my future, to hold on to.

It became a baseline to monitor my own health. I had learned to rely, to look to, the physical of my well-being, to understand what was going on underneath. I needed those dance classes as I went through my days of giving care.

The evening after diagnosis, I walked into the dance studio, a place of dusty mirrors, orange walls, battleship linoleum floors, cracking and pitted from the nails in our shoes, and a classmate asked how I was. I stared at her. I hadn't thought about what I would say if someone asked me how I was.

It didn't register with me that it was an ordinary greeting, a "hi," with no need of answer except an echoing "how are you" with no question mark. After staring at her for a moment, trying to process, saying nothing, I walked out of class. The teacher, Bev, followed me to my car, and I mumbled something to her, about how I couldn't be there that night, and drove home. Maybe I should quit, I thought, as I drove home with music cranked. I needed energy to focus; earlier in the day, I'd cancelled all my volunteer work. I'd felt a need to cut anything that seemed extraneous.

The following night, I walked back in, buckled my Seville shoes, and applied their nails to that linoleum. Bev was an intuitive teacher; did she know that the Grade 1 syllabus was perfect for me that night? Simple clapping? Basic steps? Enough to steady my mind, not so much to rattle? She knew, I'm sure. I continued with classes, as often as possible, until I could not. In October, friends in Marty's golf foursome, volunteered to stay with him while I danced, and this gave me a handful of months, so that I didn't have to give it up until the end of January, at which point I couldn't leave him with others.

Before all that, that class in June, just after diagnosis, I scratched into my journal that I didn't want to spend two hours in a class that pushed at me to focus in the way that dance does. Focus is both the gift and challenge of dance. But I went anyway. In that first class, after June 1, my inability to focus was clear, even if nothing else was. My half step behind all morning told me something. It became my baseline. I paid attention, and was gentle with myself.

Marty went to the local hospital mid-September to ascertain his baseline of breathing: lung capacity. He came home and said he "failed" the test. Something about a gag reflex. I swore it was the last test he'd go to without me. I didn't make the connection, at that point, of his baseline, and mine, in dance. That came later.

In November, his baseline was revisited when we returned for a comparative test with a respirologist who referred to his abdomen as "tummy." (We did have a chuckle about that on the way home that day. But the specialist was a Brit and also managed to crowbar "Jolly well!" into regular conversation, so had to be cut slack.) In the preliminary prep, before the measuring of more breathing (and more gag reflex and again more failure), they measured and weighed my spouse, and he was found to be three inches shorter than his 5'7" and 14 pounds less than his usual 140.

My own tummy—gut—dropped at that bit of baseline news. I recalled reading that once a patient loses 10 percent of body mass, the result is a quick decline in health.

Another dance class, Bev asked us for names of those who planned to join the studio performance at the Pacific National Exhibition. She looked at me expectantly, and I had to say, "No, I won't be able to do that." That was a first; I usually challenge myself. The "No" felt so odd in my mouth. But I needed to learn about No. Baseline.

Eight weeks later, another Saturday morning, looking in the mirror in the way that you do in a dance studio, where as an observer you see yourself: Is your arm just so, with the requisite "broken bones" of flamenco? Is your clavicle open? What's going on with your foot? Already by then, Marty could hardly turn over in bed, had given up teaching guitar, and had to frequently repeat his speech.

Looking at myself in the mirrors that morning, I had an awareness that cut me in two: that I could move, I would be able to move, and he would not. It struck me how one can "know" information, absorb it on some mental level. Then absorb it all over, knowing it in one's being. Fewer words involved, maybe none, but the knowledge penetrates, is felt. That could hurt.

By the end of January, into February, I knew I could no longer go to class. Once I'd somehow mastered the art of catheterization and feeding-tube-negotiation and deter-mining what meds and how much—a veritable Lady with the iPhone-flashlight—no one else could do what I could. For once. That did not include dance class, and was not a good feeling.

97

End of January—a Glimpse of Daily Routine

IT WAS STILL dark when we awoke. Or awoke the first time.

There'd be a half-night's worth of pee in the urinal. A full night's worth was too heavy for Marty to hold. I might have to make a quick exit, and empty it. Sometimes I picked it up, and could just feel that it would be too heavy for him. I couldn't both hold him up and hold the urinal for him.

We began the day with me pushing him, from his back, up into a semi-sitting position, and then running around to his side of the bed to pull him to standing position so we could use gravity to help him go. He'd try to stand as long as he could, but it was now only for seconds, and then I had to hold him. But hold loosely for him to navigate the urinal, and to be able to feel he could still breathe; my hold could not be tight.

If I desperately needed another ten minutes of shut-eye, I'd tuck him back into bed, careful to lay his torso only so far before bringing up his legs (or "saucering" as Ole would say, which always brought a look that we knew to be a smile), a back and forth motion, top and bottom. This process had been learned by trial and error, some pain on his part, and anxiety on mine. I adjusted his hips on one side, placed a small pillow between his knees, to relieve any pain. Tucked blankets over carefully—the blankets had to be lightly drawn over in a single layer for minimal weight, and yet had to cover to keep cold air from coming in. Always, weight was an issue. ALS muscles are tired.

But for the most part, Marty wanted to get up when he wanted to. It was not comfortable staying in bed, not with the hours he spent through the day lying and sitting.

As I went through our routine, I talked aloud about the next step. "Okay, the seat is here... right where we need it... and I'm going to lower you into it... just like that... and go around behind... up the ramp... we'll go get some breakfast ..." I did this without thinking about it. It was something I'd done with my babies, I realized. With some semi-conscious thought about language acquisition, perhaps. More, with my own need to communicate with another human.

That particular day, end of January, I suddenly felt self-conscious of this urge, this running commentary thing, and I paused to wonder what it was about. But turned out it was a bit like stopping in the midst of a trapeze act, wondering what the net was for. Madness. Because the moment I stopped talking and began to only do, I realized the issue with not talking through: As I was angling the walker into a space to catch his bum in its seat, and stopped the commentary—we'd done it so many times before, surely he knew what was next—he was suddenly nervous as I lowered him. Did he really not know what I was about to do? I was not going to drop him. I'd always gotten the angle just right; his bum met the walker seat, I pulled it in tight, or pulled him on a towel, as I'd learned to do, and I had control over this.

Hell, I had control over everything—didn't he know that by now? Without me speaking and adding words, words, words. But it turned out that the words were indeed that net for our trapeze act, and without them, there was no sense of what was going to happen next. And in our silent morning, that one day, his eyes suddenly went round and wild as if he really believed I was going to let him fall. His terror made my gut wrench.

I began to talk again, to put our net back in place, with the words I muttered all day, half to myself, half to him. I was mistaken in thinking that my chatter had no value, that it bored him.

It was a mistake I would not make again. I had to remind him I'd never let him fall. He was in tears.

Once on the walker seat, I tried to remember to switch on his computer, so it'd be ready to go post-breakfast. Then we headed for the bedroom door. I opened both doors, bedroom and to hallway, and turned on the light. I pushed him out, then backed around so I was pulling him up the ramp. I remembered to crank the furnace higher as I passed by the thermostat so when we got out of the shower it'd be warm—he was so cold always unless he was under the vintage electric blanket his cousin brought over for him. Always thinking ahead thus—or trying to—was a big part of my work. Though too often my mind emptied, and pieces escaped me.

In the bathroom, he would take a seat on the toilet. After toileting, I moved him to the shower commode, which we'd now had for almost two weeks. I'd learned that I must remember to put on the front wheel brakes... or it wouldn't be good. I lifted a side arm of this chair. (Whoever designed

it thought of everything.) I put him in, and he scrooched—
I couldn't say "scooted" because he could no longer scoot—
back, with me pushing one knee, then the other.

I put his teeth in a mug with cleaner and hot water. I
put towels on the towel rack, warming over the heat duct.
I tried to remember to leave the set of clothing on this rack
too, as it was so much more comforting to pull on warm
sweats and socks. These I left on the bottom of the pile so
they were warm after we were done. It was all this minutiae
that made a difference in the day. Perhaps it might speak to
how he was loved, even as it created physical comfort—as
much as possible.

At some point I went to the kitchen, set up coffee, and
the heating pad under the table for his cold feet. If I'd had
time the night before, I made an effort to have the oatmeal
soaking with "constipation stew" on stove, ready to have
the element turned on. Earlier in January, he'd decided to
stop the vegetable juice and most of the supplements. When
I prepared breakfast beforehand, it made all the difference;
otherwise it took forever, and if he was hungry there was a
certain impatience with the added layer of physical discomfort. What did it take for an ill person to have patience? In
the hospital, so many waited too frequently for the simplest
piece in their day. To get to the toilet, for a single Tylenol, a
glass of water, a straw.

Part of pre-shower prep was a piece of medical tape. I
removed the velcro belt that held the PEG tube, and taped
it, gently, to his chest.

Showering was the next step. I pushed the chair in under
the shower after preheating and testing the water. I had
to make certain I didn't accidentally knock the faucet and

change the temperature. (I did this once—it was not good.) I started by shampooing with just a dot. Somehow, day after day (and we did shower every day until the last ten days, when we did every second day), the moment I put the shampoo in my hand calmed me, reminded me to slow, to take all the time I had. It was the one time of day when the clock seemed to stop, and I breathed easier. He loved to have his head massaged, and his scalp was a part of his body that was pain-free. So I lathered the shampoo in my hands and took my time. Morning after morning, it was a time of reset. The night was gone, and with it the sleeplessness, the demands and misery on his part, the exhaustion and ensuing peevishness on mine. No, the exhaustion was still there, but the sun was up, and that made it different. It was time to start the clock again.

After the shampoo, I soaped everywhere. He did most of his own shaving as long as he could, which was good. Some independence. Some sense of personal care still being exactly that.

This was a longish piece of morning. The freedom of not having clothing, the joy of being—for a time—with the right temperature. The sensation—the touch and sound—of water. I too was hungry for the breathing, the contemplative feel, and so I held the water, the hose with the showerhead, moved it over him, studied what it did, studied him, his body. I thought about our past together, what he meant to me. When my mind went ahead to what the day might hold, I pulled it back into that moment. I focused on the splashing sounds, the way the light shone from the cream-coloured tiles. The way his eyelids closed with the warmth, the sensation. In the early days of assisting showering, I would be in a state of undress myself, not wanting to get my clothing wet. But several weeks of that proved too cold, and I began to wear sweats, and they got splashed and I hung them to dry afterward. The sensuality of the task was then lost for my part. But I appreciated this time for him, and we emptied the hot water tank each morning as he took some pleasure.

After, I pulled the chair to the edge of shower, and emptied water off the wide arm rests, and tried to mop up the worst. The wet floor was dangerous. I draped him in two towels, warmed over the heat. I muttered something about him looking like the Emperor in *Star Wars*, for a laugh. We could laugh about the same things over and over. I was grateful he could see the humour.

I still had to clean the feeding tube area, just above his navel, and dry it carefully, slipping gauze around the soft plastic bits that held it in place. It still amazed me, more than two weeks later, how this worked, how the human body could be met and connect with a mechanical bit such as this, and not utterly rebel. Only once had it looked a bit irritated. I'd take the gauze out before I dressed him, once I knew it really was dry. Replace his teeth as quickly as possible so he felt better and could talk. Antiperspirant. Don't forget, I reminded myself. Sometimes I did, and he didn't like that. But it grew increasingly difficult to apply once his left shoulder was in constant pain.

I moved him to the walker seat, drying drying drying the floor. Baseball shirts were the best choice at that point, with short sleeves, their roominess, the ease of front buttons; just a few nights before would be the last of putting him through the agony of pulling off a T-shirt.

When it was time to dress him, I was glad for the warmth of the clothes from the heat duct. They were cozy. Sweats or flannel jammy bottoms. Dr. Scholl's fluffy socks with sticky bits on the soles. As of a week and half before, I had to gently pull loose the toe area because otherwise it hurt his toes. Next an oversized cardigan. The best was an old XL from Cleve. Tops went first on his sore arm, and then I stretched them around to his "good" arm—though was it really much better? It was so much trial and error, and some pain in discovery. There was nothing quick about it.

At last, I wheeled the walker out to the kitchen table. Coffee and oatmeal. The heating pad under his feet made him feel good, and I tried not to forget it. I would scoop up the iPad, glasses, and phone for him.

After breakfast—and it was slow to eat—it was time to return to the studio. He'd gone through a range of spoons at that point: first spoons with foam tubing to grasp, then a welder friend actually twisted a 90-degree angle into a couple of spoons. But in short order they were too heavy, and I found a plastic spoon on a website, and ordered it.

Studio time meant moving his phone and glasses, making sure his vapourizer was there. That heating pad. Eventually, I'd get around to filling the glass measuring cup with water, and taking the syringe and a cloth and giving him his 60 millilitres of water through his tube, times four, making sure I closed and opened the tube with the clip the nurse had given us. This was his first "flushing" of the day, to keep the tube in good order for when we really needed it.

I took the time he spent at his desk, communicating with the outside world via computer, playing Scrabble on Facebook, to make the bed, do the laundry, and clean. Every morning this routine, and every afternoon another, and every evening yet another. Sister Martha in overdrive, pizza-flinging and... what was the word from the old King James Version... right, cumbered about much... too much.

I finished putting the bed together, and neared his desk to grab and empty the waste basket. As I picked it up, all the momentum of the morning came to a halt. I looked at his gnarled hands, clawing letters onto his keyboard, so slowly, his back bowed over. When had his hair gotten so thin? I could see the scar at his crown, from where he'd fallen on the front patio in the fall.

Some monstrous pang made me want to crawl back into the minutiae of the day, as it was the only way, too often, to keep moving.

98.

Guitar Notes

I step into the storeroom for something and
for the briefest moment
am taken back in time as I hear
guitar notes
a sound I haven't heard in months—
It is only YouTube

but it's last days in January and
Marty's ability to stand is going
Through this day, we both break down
so many times
grieving

Where is that growing closer
people still talk about?

I feel further and
further away

99.

Back Up

SO WHILE THE actual muscles of the bowels and bladder aren't affected, enough of the muscles around are, so the end result is an inability, or at least slowness, to eliminate effectively. With the result that urine might even back up into the kidneys. Which meant I needed to learn to wield a catheter.

I recalled a time in my young life when I avidly read those Cherry Ames books and Florence Nightingale biographies, and envisioned myself as a nurse. But that was a short-lived time and had more to do with my love of reading. And I could think of things to do with a penis that had nothing to do with finessing a thin tube inside it.

Another home care nurse came by early in the day. I warned her that I struggled to administer even nasal spray effectively, and she looked alarmed. Though she quickly said that I should be able to get the hang of it. But she admitted she had little experience with ALS. In demonstrating to me, she asked Marty to cough; he had to tell her—via text—that he couldn't really cough. He couldn't blow his nose, I let her know. You'd be amazed at the muscles you need for things you never think about.

Later, as I was poking the end of the catheter into a package of lube, Marty laughed. So did I. So did the nurse. The absurdity of it.

It took some days, and no less than three house-trips on the part of this nurse to make this happen. Dr. K mentioned trying it with Marty sitting up; he was full of tricks, our doctor, the advantage of being past retirement age. It worked, and I felt a strange sense of victory—as I did each time I confronted something that terrified me. Even if I'd never had to seriously consider the existence of certain things. Such as catheterization. I knew that *if* I had, it would have terrified me. Yet there I was, an expert.

100.

Wishes

ONE MORNING, LATE January, I received a text from Marty, asking me if I'd let "Doc"—as he called him—know about his wishes to die. He'd asked about this earlier, in the hospital, after having the feeding tube installed. He hadn't brought it up since.

I went into the studio. He texted, I talked. I asked him what was in his mind, about this. Two weeks earlier, he'd managed to speak and say, "I can't talk," as his reason for wanting not to be alive. Now he texted: *I can't do anything.*

I realized that on some level, I'd been preparing for this. My heart, taking this in, felt steadier than it had in the hospital. I had to think that he wanted to die soon, and that I had to take him seriously.

At that point in time, February 6 was the date in Canada for grandfathering such requests, with early June set as the agreed-upon date for full legalization. But I'd read the new legislation, and for people with ALS and diseases where communication was at issue, it was still a mess. There was a requirement of confirmation of initial requests; how would that work? Yet I was loath to complain as the legislation was a start at least. And had so many mad people against it. At least if it went through, there was some hope for the future. Still... caught in the middle. My mind returned to the reassuring words of the nurse in the Clinic, that the end is more peaceful than we might imagine.

Our doctor had recently taken part in a national webinar on the subject, and I knew that, even with a request, we were looking at several weeks after whatever point Marty might choose.

So we communicated as best we could, navigating the surreal. I asked him the date he had in mind. Held my breath.

My birthday, he texted.

Such a rush of emotion.

His birthday was August 24.

I wanted to weep. Did he really believe he was going to still be here at that point? With how it had progressed to date? *Did* he want to be here until that date?

There was a part of me that had had April in mind for the past few weeks—only because over the months I'd gained a sense of timing from the progression of the disease. I'd said nothing to him about this. I could be wrong. But there was a trajectory. A trajectory that terrified me, but it was there, in front of me and us. I realized, suddenly, that I'd assumed he sensed something about this. Now, I knew I was mistaken.

There was another layer. Some knowledge of healing time. What would I need? Would I ever heal? And healing time for the boys, each with his own age, experience, and needs. How would that work? It all felt so complicated and hurtful, and in the midst of it was Marty, simply naming a date that made sense to him, but without the power to be able to articulate why, and with that fogged mind. I tried to ignore the selfishness in this, but honestly the thought of what could come between February stretching to August left me feeling weak. Ole had to go back to school mid-August. How would that work? I'd been assuming I'd teach again in September—even just part-time—for that slippery sense of normalcy. If that could exist again, it would look different, I knew. But my God, how I craved normalcy. I was drowning in yet another buffeting wave of my own selfishness in that.

I didn't need to teach, I told myself. Ole could go late to school. Or something. Nothing was ever the end of the world. Not after this.

But still. I couldn't shake the feeling of despair. Under all was some serious doubt that I had what it would take to get to August. Months of broken sleep. Sometimes I questioned how I was thinking. If I was thinking.

Later, I tucked him into bed for an afternoon nap, and said, "I love you." As it had been for several weeks, there was no response. I watched him for any sign, but his face was stony. How was it that I'd thought I could read his eyes, that they would always be able to communicate with me?

A WHILE LATER, I received a text that he needed help.

In the studio, he was on the floor. For some reason—a desire for independence?— he had decided to get out of bed on his own to pee. If he'd made it, it would have been a first in weeks. He'd fallen. He texted that he had been shouting, as much as is possible, for forty minutes. I wasn't clear as to why he hadn't been able to text before forty minutes passed.

The music studio was the most soundproof room in the house. Upstairs, Ole and I had been working on his studying for an exam. The laundry machines had been running. Emmett had headphones on.

Marty had the rolly-eyed look he got when he was terrified. I had the distinct feeling that he resented me for his feeling of vulnerability. I felt sick, thinking of his panic, torn with the thought of not being there as he needed me.

I wrote in my journal: *I hate this. I just fucking hate this.*

That Night

THE FIRST FRIDAY in February became That Night in my memory. A roller coaster turn it was. After using the catheter twice, thinking I'd drained him, he insisted on peeing every ten to fifteen minutes. (Later, Dr. K pointed out that while we were used to the fasciculations of Marty's limbs, this muscle action extended throughout his body, and if the bladder was doing the same—and no doubt it was—then it would lead to a sense of constantly needing to urinate.)

I was up, taking care of this throughout the passing hours. Long hours, because we'd be in bed generally by about eight. He didn't want to sleep alone, didn't want to be left alone. I would read with a small reading light before trying to fall asleep.

When I didn't understand everything he said, he listed the people he believed understood his speech better than I. I didn't tell him that at least one of those people had told me that he smiled and nodded and pretended when they communicated. Pretence was a luxury I did not have; in order to care for him, I needed to know what he was saying. My anxiety-stopped ears needed to hear. What would it take to open them, I wondered, frustrated with myself.

That night, my loving resolve was rapidly devolving into something else. He moaned constantly, and the sound was distressing. Something beyond my understanding was spiralling out of control.

Finally, after three in the morning, he suggested we go to the living room so he could sit in his chair. For the sake of doing something, I agreed. It made sense; he could breathe with more ease sitting up.

By February, he was at the point where I had to be careful trying to get him in and out of bed, as his upper body could topple with lost balance, and he couldn't control it— although he could still sit in a kitchen chair or on the toilet once he was upright. It was just that if he started to topple, there was nothing he could do to stop it, and he couldn't warn me in time.

As I gently pulled him into a seated position that night, wrapped a light robe around him, I realized he was shivering, his entire body, with his left arm clutched to his side. I was used to dealing with his left shoulder, and the dislocation that was the result of the loosening muscles. That was bad enough. But this—this was something new. His elbow appeared to be atrophied. I tried to talk with him, to gain some sense of where he was at, and it seemed as if his speech was suddenly and thoroughly gone.

Something in my core grew cold. I couldn't understand anything he was saying. His face twisted, his eyes bulged. I tried to get another layer of clothing onto him, to warm him. Dressing him took too long, with his left arm like that, and he held his elbow so close to his body. I was certain I hurt him as I tried to pry it just far enough to pull the sleeve on. I moved him to the seat of the walker, and he slumped so much more than usual. Cold fear turned a desperate edge.

Eventually, we got to the living room, and into his big chair. I had to wake up Ole to help with this. Once in the chair, Marty fell asleep for a bit. Which was a relief. I lay on the couch and watched him, sitting there in his chair, in his Christmas gift Blue Jays shirt, and felt overwhelming sorrow well up and flood from my core to my fingertips. It occurred to me that perhaps he had experienced a stroke. Really? On top of all else? It would explain the sudden utter lack of speech, the further slackening of his face, the tightening of his limbs. While ALS had its cruise control nature, this all seemed to have taken a sudden turn that spurned the trajectory.

Yet when I discussed with the nurse the following day, she said she'd checked in with those who might know enough to have an opinion, and they felt it was the progression of ALS.

In less than a week we took over the living room as our space to sleep. When the occupational therapist ordered a hospital bed for us, Marty tried it. But he couldn't stand lying on it for longer than a half minute, before asking for his chair. For the weeks that followed, he slept in the Archie Bunker chair, upright or semi-reclined, and I slept beside him, on that bed, and left the cold leather couch.

There was no going back after That Night. Not that there ever was.

The day and night following That Night were surreal, with Marty sleeping throughout the day, utterly still. My parents came to visit, and seemed to tiptoe, said little. The house had an unusual stillness, a foreshadowing. Much as I disliked the usual noise, this was unnerving.

The day after that, however, returned to the pace of change I'd grown used to, and back to the descent.

WE GATHERED TOGETHER that Sunday to watch movies or binge on a television series—I can't recall. Something planned by Cleve. The boys reminisced and recalled how their dad used to flick them in the head to get their attention or make a point. In the next moment, they were laughing. Hard. Marty was laughing, too. We could no longer hear him laugh, but we knew he was, and it was good. If a day passed without such a laugh, I'd root around in my mind for something that might amuse. Or listen to the conversation around me for any opportunity. It distracted me, too. Mostly, it meant so much to know he had a moment away from all this. Anything for such moments of escape.

102

Too Close

AFTER A PARTICULARLY hard night of needing adjustments every ten minutes or so, I could not think what day it was. Just another morning, mid-February, ninth month in. Was it the day that Daryl came to shower Marty? It had been about two weeks at that point of having this fellow come in three to four mornings per week to spend an hour showering Marty—a retired musician, now caregiver, and able to make Marty feel at ease. We'd met him decades before—Marty had sold him backing tracks for performing—and now, coincidentally, he was reconnected by a mutual friend. These times of assisted bathing were the breaks in my week.

Marty thought it was Tuesday, and I had a moment of panic with this, because I was certain it was Monday. I said nothing, of the day or my panic.

We'd been at the kitchen table for some time, and I'd prepared breakfast, and had tried to settle Marty so that he'd be comfortable. My exhaustion was beyond what I'd ever experienced as a mother of three young children. Or even that other point of exhaustion in my life when I was twenty-seven, hugely pregnant, still working two days a week, and studying more than full-time credits in an honours program at university. Points in my life when I moved from task to task with the rote quality that terrified me; I was in that space again, and had been suspended there for so long that I could not stop to consider what it was all about. I was terrified to stop, terrified to stop the momentum.

But that day in mid-February, I received a text from my husband, sitting across the table from me: *I have to get out of here.*

A second text came: *I have to push back.*

I didn't understand. My first impulse—learned from experience—was that such messages were about the most straightforward daily reality. So this would not be existential but simply about table and chair.

I'd only just gotten Ole to take a break from studying for an online exam and come and help me adjust his dad for comfort at the table. Was he not okay at the table?

Next: *I just wanted pulled back*

And: *not too far*

Whatever was going on in Marty's head seemed to be really rattling him. I pulled back his chair—too far from the table, it seemed to me.

Even as he wrote: *I still too close.*

I pulled the chair farther away. Maybe it wasn't the nearness of the table, but about space to breathe.

Finally he appeared to settle, but then went texting off in another direction, one of directing me to uncover him in the morning. Which I thought I'd been doing. But it appeared not.

I kept my own texts to no more than one line each as I knew that any more and his mind would be unable to process the sheer amount of words.

Back and forth, trying to work though the ordinary. The ordinary could pile up, though, in a most unexpected way. I finally texted: *We have a lot of texts about day-to-day stuff. Sometimes it'd be nice to hear or see an "I love you." I'm seriously missing that.*

It was more than one line. I could have spoken aloud. But my hold on everything was so tenuous in that moment, that if I spoke the words, I'd fall apart. I sent them to the man sitting right at the table with me, and waited.

His response: *I have to poo.*

I burst into tears. Stood up. Used all my strength to pull him off the chair, and deposit him on the seat of the walker. Used all my strength and more to remind myself to be gentle. Because I did not feel like being gentle. I wheeled him to the bathroom, and set him on the toilet. *Don't just drop him. Even if you feel like it.*

I left him on the toilet and retreated to the kitchen, head in my hands, at the table. I reminded myself to breathe. Slowly. But I just sobbed.

My phone sounded. *I love you*

Another: *With all my heart*

It was the last time he said that to me. I wouldn't push at him again like that. I knew I'd prefer for it to come from him, without my push. And the sense of release and anger in me was too much.

The doorbell rang—Daryl was there.

Monday.

No pleasure in being right.

103.

Valentine's Day

I LEARNED THAT a former guitar student of Marty's died this day, a young man who not only loved rock and roll, but who also loved to fish. He was fishing in the Chilliwack River, and was dragged under when his waders filled with the cold water. I never did tell Marty. I couldn't take the thought of adding yet another layer to the sadnesses in him.

The morning after I learned of this was the first and only morning I did not awake with an instantaneous knowledge of our reality. My first thought that morning—they must have been in my dreams—was of the young man and his mother, and what his mother must be feeling. My heart wrapped around this thought and made my breath short; so hard even to allow myself to think about.

EMMETT SANG IN performance, and we both had to miss it. Cleve went, filmed it, and sent it to us.

I found Marty the next morning, sitting as he did on the toilet, with his walker in front of him to prevent falling forward, his phone in his hands, watching our youngest sing "My Funny Valentine." When it came to an end, he poked at the play arrow, and watched it through again, seemingly unaware of the tears sliding down over his face. Or unable to wipe them.

104.

You Stink

WAS IT JUST two weeks before that Marty could stand—
though only for seconds—with my arms around him, when
he woke up in the middle of the night to pee? Now he sat
on the side of the bed, and I put a robe loosely over his
shoulders, and supported him, and either he or I pressed on
his bladder to help. It needed all the help it could get. The
mechanical nature of the human body amazed me, even as
other layers, far more complicated, were at work.

That time of standing together, naked in the middle of
the night, holding him upright, now seemed so far in the
past. As we found new ways to deal with changes, the past
became a place, a series of places, we would never be again.
Suddenly those moments of standing in the murk, one arm
around his shoulders, the other supporting his lower back,
maybe a hand on his ass, now seemed to have had an odd
intimacy to them now that we were here, in a new time,
with the next step of discovering what worked as his body
changed. I now sat beside him as a helpful nurse might.
A hopeful nurse.

My biggest challenge was to feel balanced and loving. The only way I could do that was to cat nap at every possible point.

The next biggest challenge—or competing—was to understand what he was saying, and to remember what sounds meant what. What the sounds might mean the next time I heard them. I relied heavily on texting.

One morning, Marty wrote to say he'd like it if I were to get up in the night with him.

The words stunned me. I finally pointed out that I had been up every fifteen minutes or so all night. His face was utterly impassive—from the disease, but to what degree from choice, too? From ALS-messed brain? I could not know.

He wanted the television on before I'd had one sip of my coffee. My breakfast didn't have a chance. The day before, it was noon before I ate. That day my right arm was a mess, shoulder, elbow, wrist exhausted, and feeling no strength whatsoever. The lack scared me; I needed to be strong.

I longed for any expression on his face. We'd watched our wedding video in the past week, during a visit from my sister-in-law, and it was good to remember how he used to be able to express so much with a twitch of muscle, eyebrow, or quirk of mouth.

He had developed this sound that I knew to be a derisive laugh, and I dreaded it. It became a bad review of things I did that didn't rise to some standard. It was in lieu of so many words, now that spoken language was gone.

It was late in the day, nearing dinnertime, when Ole and I retrieved him from the bathroom where he'd been taking his time. We repositioned him in the chair, and I leaned over him, straightening the blanket and the pillow, as he tapped into his phone.

My phone let me know the text was to me, and I read it. *You stink.*

I had to check the rush of anger in me. I said nothing, though words flooded into my mind. I left the room, after telling Ole to keep an eye on his dad. If I didn't leave the room, I was afraid of what I might say and do.

I always tell my students that anger is a secondary emotion... this, when they treat it as a go-to in their storytelling and character development. "There is always something that precedes it, but what?" I say. (How often words to students echo in my own ears.)

Hurt was what preceded this anger in me. How could I be doing what I was doing, all I was doing, and this was his response?

To what degree should I let him off the hook for reasons of his impaired cognitive ability? Or was his humanity so compromised?

I stood in the shower, hot water sluicing over me, and tried to breathe, to calm. My showers were almost always late in the day now, and as quick as they could be, but today I took my time, and let anger move from boil to simmer. I would like to just let it go, but the hurt, if I stopped to feel it, was deep. Damaging. I was aware of that. At times, I was back in the time of my marriage before—back in the time of taking for granted. I didn't know how we'd gotten there. Or why the hell we'd want to be there. Not when we could be drawing strength from what we'd had in the more recent past. It seemed to me that we'd built enough from that to carry through. But it seemed now as if I was the one of us who thought this. How could that be?

How well can we know anyone?

Again, I was left pondering Marty's reality, and what it meant to be dying. And the nature of ALS, and specifically, his ALS, with its cognitive impairment. No one explained that, or even talked about it. In Clinic visits, it didn't come up—not for his perspective, or for my part in his life. I had to feel my way through it.

There was so much I couldn't know. Both about his individual experience, and the experience of dying. Text messages could not cover this ground, especially not when it was ground we'd not so much as flown over in our earlier time together.

Someday I will know more, perhaps, when I am dying myself. If a giant grand piano doesn't just drop on me, and leave me unaware—which, I was beginning to think was the way to go, for all of us.

But I wouldn't know until I got there, and my "getting there"—my being the dying—would be forever changed from what it might have been before this experience. I was reviewing this process in a way that not so many people needed to before their own time. So I had the strange advantage of that. If someone was taking care of me, would I be different? Now, after this, I might be.

Not for the first time, I wondered how we'd be in a reverse of this situation, if I were in his place, and he in mine. It was not a good place for my mind to go; I had a distinct feeling that I would be in a hospital, and he would be visiting me. As I articulated that to myself—if I articulated it—I could feel some despair welling in me. Maybe I was mistaken. Or maybe that was how it should have been. But I'd made a promise, and the promise had made sense to me. And it still did.

I had not brought my phone into the bathroom with me. I wanted freedom from it.

The shower was good. It was good to be clean and washed and human. Maybe the tyrants of our world were just short a few showers. It could do it. Going without a shower could mutate one into something less human.

I returned downstairs to where Emmett was now watching his dad, and Ole had gone to do homework, with Emmett's schoolwork on hold.

I asked Marty, trying to keep my tone light, if he intended for his text to be something of a joke—did he intend this to be a bit funny?

He stared at me.

Then typed in a message to let me know he was uncomfortable. I would have to rearrange and smooth his clothing, and the pillow and such. But before I did, I caught sight of a much earlier message from some hours ago, when I was too busy to read my phone—an earlier message also noting that I stank.

I let it all be until the following day. I needed time to calm.

The next day, at the breakfast table, I pointed out that those messages hurt. That there was a great difference between writing me such, and sending a message to one of the boys to say, "Take care of me while your mom showers."

There was a barely perceptible twitch of recognition in his face, enough to allow me to see that he understood the difference. There was still humanity—the possibility of it—between us then. I was glad I waited a day to come up with words to let him know what to do. But the consciousness of it all, the directing, was tiring.

105.

Mary

Where are you?
I can't see you kneeling at Jesus's feet. But I'm not there
either
I can't see you checking out my winter garden
or anywhere
Am I just missing you?
Are you here, right in front of me?

Can't you whisper to me to slow down? Isn't there
something you are supposed to remind me of? Can't you
shout over Martha's shoulder, and get me in line
on track?

Stop your staring at the moon
As if it has answers
Here. Take this. Do something

106

Most Sought

MY FOREARMS BOTH ached. My jaw was something I'd like to cut out of me. That tooth was still acting up—as they say. I seemed to be developing a sinus infection. In the middle of the night, I held an ice cube to my forehead and cheekbones, willing the sinus to numbness. I had pains in my left breast. The thought of being ill myself terrified me. My boys were so tough, but that would be the breaking point.

So much seemed to be pressing in and down; kindness was what I most sought through those days, hunting it, in myself and others. Trying to relieve the sense of pressure.

It was an afternoon, and Marty was napping. When he slept, his eyes were half-opened, yet when he was awake they were half-closed. Or perhaps it was the same. The radio tried to roar over the blowing and sputtering of the nebulizer, its thin plastic mask with saline mist over Marty's face. The soundtrack to my life. Moments of silence made my heart ache. But today, this afternoon, I was grateful for the coffee mug in my hands, and a moment to read. There was something so comfortable in us being side by side, napping and reading, and life slowed. I sought out as much of such time as I could.

I thought about how someday, in my future, I would need to fall in love with myself before anything else could happen. There were parts of me that I didn't much like right then; I could see them clearly. At least, I thought I could. I tried to struggle beyond this person I was revealing myself to be. I promised I'd take care of her, whatever was left.

107.

We Are Watching Television
---

the series *House of Cards*

but I am half there   the other part
of me dealing with kitchen and
dishes and sorting
bottles of laxative and
painkiller
and breakfast lunch dinner Boost for that tube

when Marty sends a text
you'r mising it

and I find my seat on the couch
look at the TV
look at him

breathe

108.

People Would
Drop By

I UNDERSTOOD. WHILE I knew that the stop at our house was an item on their to-do list, it was a significant part of their list. I could guess at the courage it took because of times in my own life when I'd either risen to or slunk away from such challenges.

Visitors would come with things in their hands. Sometimes they'd hide behind these things. When I took them from their hands, there'd be a shrinking motion on their part. The gifts might be bread—too hard for Marty to chew, would cause choking, but it was appreciated by other members of the family. Good to remember the caregivers. Or tea that he and I could share. Later, it might be bath supplies for me. Which I did make use of, if there was a boy around to keep an eye on his dad. The bathtub was a place to crawl to for respite. Sometimes people brought fruit, which was nice.

What is the nature of simply showing up? Yet invariably that was how it happened. Not a bad thing. I just mull over that choice. Too difficult to text me or get me on the phone— would that create more a sense of interrupting? Perhaps it would. Some of the folks who came by probably did not have my number or the family landline, but only Marty's number. Perhaps, calling ahead, planning, made it more formal and binding. There might be a need to back away suddenly from the decision. Did people come, sit in their car outside our home, question if they could do this thing… and then drive away? I would understand that. Later, in the program for the memorial service, I chose to place a few words about the choice not to visit, and for those who chose not to, to absolve their selves. Marty never visited people when they were ill; he struggled with it. Each person had to make their own choice about this. Several friends did not visit but sent beautiful and thoughtful cards every couple of months. I would put these on the bar that ran the length of the kitchen where I could see them throughout the day, and they strengthened me. Missives to connect with Marty. Missives from a world I would rejoin at some point.

One visitor was Mike, the musician friend we'd gone to see that first weekend after initial diagnosis. He never came for long, but he made several visits over the months. The first time he showed up looking terrified, and stayed some few minutes. The second time, again a short visit, he looked somewhat more at ease. For Marty, such visits were just long enough to break up the stretch of day. The third and last visit, though not completely at ease, Mike was more natural. I admired his resolve and friendship.

With many visitors, I came to recognize the role I subconsciously stretched to, that of a sort of docent. Docent of illness, ALS, grieving, mourning. Learning the difference between grieving and mourning helped me to navigate this in a small way. The difference guided me to distinguish between the private and the public.

Toward the end, people came, perhaps knowing or thinking it would be their last visit.

Some came from afar, and I had to tell them that they would have to stay elsewhere for their sleeping time, and that their visits must be short. Two hours at the most, not overlapping. I had to plan, and explain the overstimulated concussed quality to many, even to Marty's sister, and to an old friend, to people who had often stayed in our home as if it were a second home, as it had often been.

One morning, when I reminded Marty of the line-up of visitors for that day, he began to weep with immediate exhaustion. I contacted people and shortened their visits. I didn't tell them about the tears.

Later in the day, after a couple of earlier visits, Marty slept in his chair surrounded by my brother, sister-in-law, nephew, and his spouse. My brother had attached a soap shelf in the new shower, and my sister-in-law had set about cleaning the house—I'd had to stop her, tell her the visit was more important. She also made stew and replenished the freezer. She'd done enough. My nephew was about to vacuum upstairs. Instead we all gathered around sleeping Marty, and watched the hockey game, on low volume. It was a special game, NHL players on an outdoor arena for Canadian annual hockey day.

There was a magical quality to that afternoon, and the quiet of it, the murmured voices, the odd bit of low laughter, replenished. Marty was sleeping, surrounded by love that felt to honour this passage. They were all a bit teary and a little lost looking as they left.

109.

Food

Just shows up
In the fridge, the freezer, on the wide doorstep out
front
foil-wrapped, with a note on top
The last twelve weeks, no planning
on some anonymous person's part
yet never too much or too little. Sometimes
people say "I'll do Tuesday... except
when I'm away," and even then
it works
In that time I cook only twice—pizza
and barbecue hamburgers
two family favourites that leave me hungry
to create, but that time will come
In the meantime
this
is a miracle

110.

Trespassing

A DANCE CLASSMATE was a massage therapist, and she invited me for a massage with her. At first I said no—no time. But as my physical pain continued to deepen, I realized this was not unnecessary or an option, and I set up a time when Cleve could come by and look after his dad.

The classmate's home was in the town next to us, ten minutes away, where my parents both still lived in the house in which I grew up. The route I drove that day, to go to her house—she had an at-home spa space for her business—took me by my parents' place, and as I passed, I caught sight of my eighty-four-year-old father, strong as an ox after years of building homes, out mowing and raking his ditch. Madness, so early in the year. Why? He loved to be busy and hard-working. I saw, suddenly, that he was indeed an old man, one I had not spent enough time with lately. The thought that I would be experiencing widowhood before my mother ever did came to me. *What was that?*

On the way back home, I passed so many places and so many memories. We had lived in those small towns for almost two dozen years. I was going to now know the inside of the funeral home, I thought, as I passed it. Memories were memories even before they should be; I'd stumbled into some place marked NO TRESPASSING. There were places I just didn't need to know the inside of.

Mostly, there was the place inside me that had accepted this was happening. Was going to happen. Had happened.

My classmate, post massage, told me I was brave. Was I? Or just doing what I needed to do? Was that brave? Were there options?

turn thr heat dow

AT THE END of February, when Dr. K showed up for his weekly visit, Marty was agitated, and appeared to want to say something to the doctor. I was trying to grow more alert to the nuances of agitation—what was hunger, what was medication, was the medication for pain or anxiety. This agitation I'd seen twice before now: it was about that question. The window of time for Marty to have any control over his ability to make a call on the length of his own life was slipping; his texts were starting to take on other-worldliness, with misspellings, and gaps in comprehension.

I got the iPad for him, with its larger keyboard, and asked him what he wanted to say. He struggled to type, he deleted, he struggled again. At last the message: *turn thr heat dow*.

Really? That's what he wanted to say? So I'd misunderstood. Utterly.

Dr. K gave a wry chuckle.

I took Marty to the bathroom as it was the time of morning when we were waiting for Daryl to arrive to shower him, and I needed to prepare for that. I did my puttering, and Marty typed. *In wanna givve*. Then, a moment later: *I wanna due.*

More waiting. Then: *I wanna die.* I told him I'd speak with the doctor, and put an arm around him gently. Wished I could say more, but Daryl turned up just then. While he and Marty were in the bathroom, Dr. K and I talked together in the main room. He didn't seem to feel it was time yet. He even said something about me not being ready. Was I? Was I not? He advised me, though, not to count calories. Feed Marty when he was hungry. Medicate as much as needed. Now is the time for comfort, Dr. K said.

Marty never did question me about Dr. K's answer. And he never again brought up the subject.

112.

Yes and No

On the last day of February, I realize
I can no longer hear
any difference between his "yes" and "no."
The words sound
the same.

Daryl reports:
March 8 is the day
that Marty can't shave
even half his face

113.

Warbling

SIX TRIPS TO the toilet through one night. Each time, the results were nothing. Just a body misreporting. Urges from muscles that no longer had a director. The fourth trip, my arms began to give out as I moved him from walker to toilet seat. With whatever strength was left in them, I should lower him to the floor. Which I did, as carefully as I could, and placed towels under his head, and went to awaken Ole to help. The next trip, I awakened him first, before moving Marty.

I did come up with a way to set the walker against a wall or a heavy chair, so that I could do this on my own, and this worked, but there was the fallout of this earlier lowering-to-the-floor: Marty no longer trusted me.

I could feel the anxiety in him, and had to address it directly. I pointed out that I had not actually let him drop; that the release to the floor was careful, calculated. I understood why he felt he couldn't trust me, and apologized for that. But that he had to trust, and that I would live up to my end. He seemed relieved by the blunt talk. The acknowledging of the reality, and my part in it.

It felt as if all my life I'd watched others do this—this bluntness. It wasn't a default setting for me; it was something I had to pull out of myself. I wished, at the time, and times through the months before, that I could push and pull at him, and with myself, to have the conversations I thought we needed to have, for both our sakes. *What is happening to us? What does it mean? What can we do about it? What is it to die? What is it to live?* Questions I'd wanted to talk about for months now. But it was too late. We'd talked about what it meant to take care of him, the ins and outs, the practicalities. We'd even talked about dying, inasmuch as it meant assisted death. But we hadn't talked about what might come after and his fears or thoughts. We hadn't talked about my living, for that matter. He never brought up any of these words, not while he'd been able to speak, and not through the months of keyboard communication. It weighed on me, that this had not happened.

But perhaps equal in significance: When was the last time he laughed? I rooted around in my mind, my short-term memories, for the *when* of that. I tried to relay a story Ole had shared, about a friend of his—a big kid we had known since he was a boy—suiting up for work. It was a funny story, but it drew only a blank look, and that slow and dismissive sweep of eyelids. His cognition had dulled for details and stressful information. But it had also dulled for wit and even simple fun. I'd missed the window for serious conversation, yes, but I also missed our day-to-day ordinary sharing of stories and nothings. When I spoke now, most of the time it quickly came to an end as he flapped his hand to get my attention, and tried to let me know he needed a blanket pulled down, or pillow pulled up, or something to make the moment more comfortable. Or of less discomfort. This was what remained. Did he miss the team as much as I did?

THERE WAS A new sound to his moaning at night, a sort of warbling quality, unbearable to hear. I could not tune it out. It haunted. What was the pain he felt, with his dislocated shoulder? Yet when I questioned him about wanting a third dose of morphine in quick succession, and I asked if this was for physical pain, he indicated the "no" (red square) response on the chart given to us by the communications people. When I asked if it was about emotional pain, he indicated "yes" (green square). So perhaps the warbling was in lieu of tears. My heart stretched with more pity, and I wished that I could know what he was feeling. My own sadness was so deeply in my bones; I knew that someday I would have to try to come to an understanding of what it would take to ease the sadness out of my own self. And what, now, would it take to ease his? It did not seem possible. Those podcasts? The television? Maybe just me staying close by?

With the change to living room as sleeping space, I no longer felt isolated in the night-time airfield of Marty's studio, which had really always been his space. In the open main room of the house, I could get up in the middle of the night, heat milk, stir honey into it. Do yoga stretches. Set out yin cards, and follow their slow poses, held for minutes that allowed me to breathe and relax, almost. I could read with a low directed light over my page. These things, though momentary, made the days and nights different. It may have even allowed for us to feel close, and in that there was some respite from sadness. This room had always been a shared and family space, and in it Marty was never alone. Boys joined us for television, then left us for the night.

I thought about being a child, when sleeping in the living room meant sleeping by the Christmas tree. Living room space was magical then. I wasn't sure I would want to sleep in this room again for any reason. Something had taken over, and it was a changed space from where the boys all slept under the holiday tree. Even when the fire was lighted now. Yet, that wasn't quite fair, as it was also the social place, and a warm and welcoming part of the house... was no doubt how guests saw it.

Sometimes, I opened the curtain by the hospital bed where I slept in our living room, and watched the rain come down. The winter had been stormy outside, too, and the rain at times pounded into the windows that lined our back wall, ceiling to floor. I was grateful for this weather that reflected so much, and didn't let me think of other things I might be missing. I didn't want spring to come. I didn't want to see green peeping out, green I couldn't go out into the yard to inspect in a leisurely way.

Just close us off with the grey, and the rain, and the wind, so inside feels like where I want to be.

114.

Normal

I tell Dr. K that I seem to irritate Marty a lot of late
and he responds that this is normal:
the terminally ill have a subconscious urge
to make you hate them, is how he puts it.
"That way, you'll miss them less"

"Do you mean like when the boys and I used to spend
a summer at my brother's
and in the last 24 hours of every visit
Cleve and his cousin used to fight and almost
come to blows...
and it always made leaving easier?"

"Exactly," says Dr. K
Exactly like that

115

March On

WE PASSED MID-MARCH, the day our first son was born. Noteworthy because Marty ate a few bites of food, Cleve's birthday cheesecake. He hadn't eaten food in several weeks; he'd had only the bottled feeding tube so-called nutritional drinks, with sweetener and flavours that bypass all buds and go straight to the gut.

When Cleve came over, it was through the front door, swinging, calling out as he came, "Hey, Dad! Hello! I love you!" as if refuting the reality that Marty could not respond.

Earlier in the day, Marty had had a not-temporary catheter put in, and he was not happy about it. In the middle of the night, he moved his hand and began to pull on it as if to pull it out. The sharpness in my voice when I said, "Don't do that!" scared me—sharpness borne of the thought of yet one more night of temporary catheter routine. It was tricky getting that tube in just so, and withdrawing, often with overflow and clean-up. And too often, without result.

NIGHTS GREW MORE difficult. It seemed as if every time I began to drift toward sleep, he would need something. He could make the slightest sound to call for my attention, and I would hear. Sometimes it felt to be a call from some silent space in him to a silent space in me, and I'd be up. Once, when tired beyond anything in my experience, I told him I needed two hours, just two solid hours of uninterrupted sleep. I didn't set a timer. I also didn't think he could see the clock on the television cable box. I had no idea what his sense of time was at that point. Or if he understood my need. It was deeply into the middle of the night.

In exactly two hours and one minute, he woke me up. I had managed to fall to sleep. When I awoke at his sound, I looked at the clock, saw the time, and wondered why he couldn't let me be. I started to cry, and my tears—pressure relief valve—made me angry. Everything at that moment made me angry. Later, I tried to think if the two hours just passed was coincidence, or something innocent. But at that moment it seemed intentional and it hurt.

Another night Ole said that he would stay with his dad for the night, and I went upstairs to sleep. It was a break for me, but too much for a young person, and eventually, toward the morning, he went to bed, and I took over. But it was a break.

The local health unit sent out a professional caregiver once for a couple hours one afternoon, and I never asked for another. I spent half the time training him, and the other half making sure he did the tasks correctly. Mostly, he wanted to chat with someone about his career plans. The health unit had already let me know that it was unlikely I'd get the same person on a regular basis; that was not how they scheduled care. The thought of subsequent training and observation time did little for me.

Ultimately it came down to two choices: hospital or me. I had made a promise, and I wanted Marty surrounded by family. I had to remind myself of these choices, in the middle of the night. It wasn't until close to the end that I began to open my mind to the possibility of hospital or hospice. Unknown to me until later was the fact that Dr. K was trying to place Marty in hospice even just for a week to give me a break.

Although the boys did learn how to administer medication ("I'm giving my dad morphine!" said Emmett, once. "This is so weird!"), it was the timing, careful questioning as much as possible, and the intuitive sense of how much—and that only came with the experience of day in, day out care, and those nights.

Early on, we'd created a homemade chart with frequent requests and words on it. Later, we added the communication people's chart with colours to indicate yes/no. And this included a yellow "maybe." I recall wondering at the usefulness of that with a nurse friend; what was the "maybe" about?

On the homemade chart, the requests were straightforward, and as we worked through needs, some—written around the edges and outlined with marker-pen boxes—became very particular. His cognitive capacity, however, meant that at times he pointed to the wrong box, almost as if he had some sort of memory as to the nature of a box, but had forgotten which box it was. I remember wishing, in the last few weeks, that we'd included boxes for "Thank you!" and "I love you"—anything to soften what became little more than a series of commands and requests. Perhaps that yellow "maybe" was a softener. A couple of our worn-out joking words would have been respite, would have made me feel less utilitarian. Was he okay with his constant demands? Did he wish for something else, too? I wished I could be freed of my desire for some form of acknowledgement, or sign of gratitude.

Texting became of almost no use in the last days, and he could spend fifteen long minutes with the iPad, only to let me look at the screen and see that what he'd poked out of the keyboard resembled Welsh.

It had been months since we were able to share a hug. Now there were times I'd like just to hold his hand, or place a hand on his arm. Twice he pushed away my hand. There were nights when, in the middle of the hours, in the tending to requests, when I tried to bring some moment of warmth, he wouldn't look at me. Twice, I remember trying to move into the line of his gaze, only to have him look elsewhere. "Can you look at me?" I asked once, middle of the night. He wouldn't. Sometimes I had the feeling he was angry with me. Once I wrote in my journal—because I'd vowed that everything that went into the journal had to be my felt-truth—that it seemed as if he either wanted me to go with him, or that he felt I should go in his place. Mostly—truth—I felt the latter.

Sometimes it seemed as if we were in a small plane, going down, in a not-so-slow nose-dive, and he'd opened the door, and was deciding whether to jump or push.

I couldn't let my mind go there. But it did. Was it just sleep deprivation? I fought back the thoughts that invaded me.

IN THE LAST week, though, in spite of these shadows and miserable thoughts that hovered, a different sort of tenderness grew. It didn't feel to have much connection with marriage really. It felt raw and human. Six days before he died, he awoke in the morning with marked change to his breathing. It was even heavier, more laboured; there was a deep-sea quality to it, an absorbed, though unconscious, focus. The medication he was on—fentanyl—seemed to answer his old request for heroin if he was ever that ill. He was sleepy, with eyes never opening far, never alighting on something with recognition.

Dr. K showed up, after I called to tell him about the change in breathing. He spoke with Emmett, reassured him that everything was as it should be. He was speaking to me, too, I knew. He didn't seem to think it was near the end.

As I moved about the house in those few days, the feeling of tenderness and pity grew in me, in response to his breathing. It softened the edges that had been growing. And yes, it was just human.

It was that last week that I needed another set of hands— Ole or Emmett—for taking Marty to the toilet, and when Daryl came to shower Marty, I now helped him as he needed extra hands. A couple of times that week, I did so without Daryl, and I took even longer than usual, just to break up the day further, and because I imagined that showering really was the best of the day for Marty, lying back in that chair, warm water over his muscles, the sound of water, and splashing on the tile.

The tenderness felt fragile. I found myself thinking in tiptoe, not wanting to frighten it or roar it away. The feeling wrapped around all of us there in that house. In the end, I was glad this had somehow found us, washed over us, taken away some of the shadow stuff in its tide as it washed out and away in the days after he was gone. But still, the shadows were there, the sadness. The sadnesses.

116.

Weight

Bone-deep exhaustion, sinus infection full on—
so when Daryl shows up
to shower
I tell him I'm going upstairs
to sleep in what used to be my bed

This room is cold and stilled. There is laundry
piled on the side of the bed where Marty has always
slept. I don't move it
to lie down for what will be a short nap or, more likely,
nothing more
than a time of not getting up. I don't move
the laundry; I like the sensation of weight
beside me

117.

Like Some Bad

I REMEMBERED THE wish to grow old together—and we did. We just grew old before our time.

I didn't know it at the time, but we were down to our last days. I did feel we were closing in somehow. Yet there wasn't a sense of reality to that. Later, I was left with a "wish-I'd-known." The knowledge might have infused me with third-wind—or fourth—energy.

My boys and I comforted each other with hugs. Such hugs took place elsewhere in the house—in the studio, the upstairs hall, out in the sunshine on the deck—spontan-eously, after snippets of conversation, confessions of no longer wanting to see their dad as he was, or wishing they'd exchanged some words. We were strengthening, preparing. They kept me going; we kept each other going.

When I researched "restlessness" through the online uni-versity library, I read more than one article—no, I didn't read, I skimmed—about how, in last stage, people with ALS experience daytime fatigue and night-time restlessness and insomnia. That was what we were experiencing, certainly. But still. It didn't seem possible that we were close to the end.

In the last week, diapers became a reality. The community health nurse brought them, showed me how to use them, in the event I had any questions. Not likely.

One of Marty's golf-mates came around. He had visited weekly at the least, often took my place while I went to dance class, and being the cook in his family, had taken to bringing us homemade dishes since the fall.

But now, diaper advent, he felt it incumbent to talk with the friend he considered his closest. Coincidentally, this friend had been diagnosed with Parkinson's just six weeks before Marty's diagnosis.

We didn't realize then that it was The Last Day. Or last full day, anyway. While I gardened and pretended to think about other things, Marty's friend sat with him and the Yes/No/Maybe chart, and tried to ascertain his end-of-life wishes. The time together stretched to more than an hour. Apparently, Marty's hand hovered to the Yes, then the No, then the Yes. Maybe a Maybe was in there, too. This went on.

Finally, the friend threw up his hands. "Man," he said, "you are like some bad Ouija board!"

That would have brought out a full-on laugh from Marty at another time in his life.

118.

Grace

I HAVE YET to be the one who is dying, and it's possible that I'll feel differently when I'm on that side of the coin. But I hope to remember. To have some grace. What is grace? I grew up with the word. When I let my gut define it, I feel that grace is an openness, a softness, a kindness. Something merciful. There's another good word. Dictionaries use the word "unmerited" to describe the definition that is concerned with grace as divine assistance. That word makes me pause, because it takes "grace" to another level. Unmerited. To me, that speaks of reaching more deeply even into whatever resources I may have had and not had. I did my human best. But it was lacking. I knew that. I like to think sleep would have helped, that it was that simple. I've had a wish to go back to that time, to have a re-do, but with sleep, to see what kindness there might have been. I hope there would be more.

Somehow, life and death need to be lived and experienced through the lenses of these words—grace and mercy. I know that. But it may well require "divine assistance."

Will I remember grace when I am dying?

I am now in a place of watching my parents go through what I have already been through, an odd thing indeed. (My father was diagnosed with ALS the following December. Two random, "sporadic," incidents within a family and suddenly the disease does not seem so rare.) The situation seems to be different because they are thirty and more years older than I at the time I went through. Energy levels are different. My father's ALS has left his mind as clear as ever, unlike the cognitive challenges Marty faced, and began with his speech, breathing, eating, rather than in his hands, where Marty's symptoms began.

Sometime after Marty died, I was speaking with a woman who told me a story that stayed with me, about a couple she knew, a late middle-aged couple, with a strong marriage that still held a double dose of romance.

When the woman was diagnosed with a life-threatening illness, the husband committed to caring for her. With a caveat: he would never wipe her ass. "She's my *wife*," the person telling this story recalled. "That's what he said. He'd never wipe her ass. It couldn't be part of the deal." The deal being the fragile business of why we choose to marry a particular person.

I'm not convinced this story would have meant much to me at the outset of my own time of caregiving. But at the end, just weeks after Marty was gone, I wished, desperately, that someone had related it to me years before. I wished I'd had the time to absorb it, to have taken it on. Really, I wished I'd thought of it myself. How had that not happened? How did I grow so overwhelmed that I couldn't come up with this most obvious boundary? The sense of being overwhelmed cut off so much rational thought—even the most ordinary.

There hadn't seemed to be boundaries when I signed up. That is, given that I was relatively young and strong, and could take leave from my job, the path seemed possible. I knew there would be challenge and sadness and pain. But I did sign up; I responded to what felt to be a call of life and love. I'd felt like something of a hero, going in. The hero, boarding the plane, about to take off, waving to those below. At the time it seemed to be more about honouring my partner, my marriage. It seemed to be the thing to do, really. That simple.

Early on, in those first one hundred hours, it seemed to be the least I could do. In no small degree, it was something of a go-to place for me. And it had all the romance of a call to arms. I can't deny that. God knows, I wanted to hold on to romance, in any way. Like most calls to arms, there was death and sacrifice, and too much of both.

I never considered the cost of wiping a beloved's ass.

Truth is, I'd gladly wipe an ass if I thought the receiver of the wiping could find a way to accept, to look me in the eye afterward, would let me hold his hand—after a good wash, of course. I'd also gladly wipe if I knew he'd wipe mine. Dogs meeting and greeting in their way begins to almost make sense.

I'm being facetious because humour is necessary to my well-being. But really the ability to take on new roles is imperative—to slip in and out of either Martha or Mary and to suspend judgement on which is more significant or needed. Maybe there's even a beauty or a particular love to ass-wiping, something I've missed.

We can't know. Until we are there. Not even then. I only wish that each of us could remember to take the time—no, I wish we could *have* the time (so challenging to take what we don't have)—to reflect, to know our mind and needs in order to do what is asked of us. But often, mostly, when life asks much of us, such time cannot be had. In John Bayley's memoir, about his beloved wife, Iris Murdoch, who lived with Alzheimer's, he writes of how she used to go out and collect bits and pieces from the street, and these—garbage, essentially—accumulated in their home, and he lived with it, and knew that the presence of a house-cleaner would be distressing to her.

I ponder how collecting whatever it takes to build resilience throughout our lives might be analogous. We may be the only ones knowing what it is we need, but it is important that we go out and glean our bits, bring them in, so that when the time comes, we have what we need to get through. The word "knowing" may go too far; we generally don't "know," but even to gather together elements of our world that resonate with us, that feel to have the capacity to build and strengthen us, to do this in healthy times, will surely grow and feed us in times that are not healthy. Such elements might not make sense to another, but we might have some nebulous sense of their worth. Or trust that they are necessary for us.

I scribbled words in the middle of the night, as an image of childhood musical chairs came to me: *you are left holding in your hands whatever you had at the moment the music stopped.* Whatever you have built of your life at the moment you receive diagnosis, there it is. Your basket of food with which to create your last feast. You can't go back into the garden to gather more. But out into the wilderness. That's how it seemed to me. We collect experience, we connect with others, we build laughter and soul and home—so that when we need a foundation and a shelter, it will be there for us. But if it hasn't been built, the sand under us will give way. The phrase "too late" came to my mind at moments, despairing moments, through the months. Still, I didn't want to give up. I couldn't.

In my one term of teaching, in the fall that Marty was ill and I was caregiving as many hours as I could—teaching time and grocery store trips being the only exceptions to time with him—I would look out at the young, tired, hopeful, resigned faces of 260-some second-year students taking my introduction to writing for children class, and I would wonder. First, what sort of teacher I was that term. Quick answer to that one: I knew I was not my usual. (Why was I there? Habit. Normalizing.) Second, how much to tell them. (Little: My spouse has ALS. You might see more of your teaching assistants and guest-speakers than you see of me this round.) Third, I wondered about them, and worried. Mental well-being is such an issue on campuses. Young students are unable to keep up with deadlines and pressures. When I make provocative statements such as, "Don't worry! This isn't the real world!" they look at me, stricken. *This* is Everything, they've been told. Their Entire Future Depends on This. "You have no idea," I want to say. This is just building who you are for what is to come.

Challenge is opportunity. Build. Grow. And as Patti Smith has said, "Love each other, motherfuckers!" Everything depends upon that, and maybe that alone, at the end of the day. Forget the white chickens and the red wheelbarrow. It's not an inactive or quiet love. There's an active *doing* urgency—even anger—to Smith's words.

Love one another so fiercely it begets its own energy.

119.

Midday, Sunday

April 10, 2016
I remember

The sun was shining
It was a slow day to begin with. He was quiet
all morning
Fentanyl? Or knowing the time had come?
I'd turned off the television—tired of golf Masters—
and turned on Steely Dan

as he always wanted
After all that
it seemed so sudden

Neighbours came with fully cooked dinner
We sat around the fire

Wind chimes
I slept in my own bed.

120.

Flamenco Revisited

IN THE CURIOUSLY lightened state of after-care, I had to find a way to kick-start a new normal. The booklet given to me by the funeral home folks called this state "euphoric." It was not that. I'll stay with "curiously lightened."

Tuesday class-time, I was in the funeral home signing papers.

But Wednesday night came. I put on my skirt. Shoes, castanets, and fan were in their dusty bag. I took them to the car.

And sat in the driveway. *Can I go?*

Would I remember steps? My muscles might. But would my soul?

My skirt hung loosely. Would it swing? Calf muscles ached, shoulders were tight from lifting and setting down with care. Too many nights of not sleep but naps.

What was left of me now? What was left to me? Did I want to know?

Would there be joy in my *bulerias*? Maybe just sorrow in *solea*.

My flamenco teacher, Bev, would drill us on errant body parts and missteps. "Application!" she would say. "Apply what you have learned!"

We live, we learn, but can we apply... when the application closes in on terror?

In the rapid terror-filled progression of Marty's ALS, there was no time for application. Or so little time.

But I still felt a need to create noise in my flamenco cave. That was still inside me, I discovered, as I sat there in my car, in my driveway. For now, that was what I would do. Or try.

There was a sense of wondering how I'd come to be where I was: in my car, going to flamenco class. So normal. So not. A sense of blindly with clear eyes going forward, hoping to God that life would catch up somehow. And when it did, it would find me living.

Tammy (the friend who'd helped with the question of when and how to tell the boys) had told me never to turn down any offer of help. In the early days after Marty passed, I determined that I would never say no to an invite—whether a friend-invite, or a life-invite—to connect with others, to dance, to hear music. I would not hide away.

I turned the key. I drove to dance class.

121.

Viewing

AT WHAT POINT after that Sunday was I told that I needed to come in to the funeral home on the fourteenth, Thursday? They needed me to identify the body. Or I could give them a picture, was an option.

After I saw my father-in-law's body, the only I'd ever seen to that date, I promised I would not intentionally view a dead body again. But this was different. Not sure how. Maybe it was having gone through so much, that to see this path to its end—and this seemed to be some part of the end—was significant. I said I'd be there. "You can change your mind," the funeral home director reminded me.

Others could come too, he added. But I went alone. On Wednesday, late, a thought came to me, as I was considering the necessity of doing this. It occurred to me that it might be good to see Marty's body at rest. Those first times of seeing the fasciculations in his arm, feeling them under my fingertips, feeling the horror of it, even as it slowed in the later months of the disease, indicating the neurons were dying, didn't diminish the revulsion and anger I'd felt. Now to see his body at peace might mean something.

Always looking for meaning.

So I went.

The stillness to a funeral home. The solemnity. A business trying to appear to be something else.

"Take your time," said the woman seeing me to the door of the family viewing room.

Once again, alone, stepping through the door, I questioned: Is this me, here, doing this? Looking at my husband's body? Saying some other type of goodbye?

Reminding myself, this was the last time I would ever see this man's body. The body I had come to know in these months in ways I'd never before known. Ways I'd never thought I'd know.

From the doorway, I could see the crest of his forehead, and as I neared, the side of his face. I was ready to exit quickly. But it wasn't necessary; there was a strangely natural feeling to this, so different from viewing his father twenty-two years before. I had a familiarity with this body that made this work. That made it necessary.

Through my mind flashed my promise to keep him at home, and my nurse-friend's words: "You didn't know what you were promising." Words she spoke two days before he passed.

His eyes were closed. Some part of me wondered how they achieved that. Crazy glue? What a thought. I recalled Marty telling stories of guitar players, crazy-gluing their fingernails if they broke them in music school. How many stories would it take to get me through this? Was I going to remember them? Would they drift from me? Would they drift away before I shared them with the boys?

I went closer. His hands were gently cradling each other, like a yoga mudra I'd used often to comfort myself. I reached into my pocket for a guitar pick I'd found and brought with me, and now placed it inside the curve of his fingers. The golf clothes, with the shirt from his club, looked good. His chest was so thin, like a child's. I'd never noticed that it had come to look like that. Somehow the slackness of ALS wasn't so much in his face now, though, and he was shaved smooth. There was a calm. Finally. So good to see.

I told him I'd talked to an estranged friend. That the friend had shared how much he'd cared for him. I told him the plans were going all right for the service. I told him we'd be all right. We really would be. (Would we? I questioned.) Really, we would be. I told him I loved him. I told him his voice and words would be with me.

That's when I realized: My spouse was gone. But my marriage was still with me. My marriage was with me until I decided it wasn't. That was in my control. This thought strengthened me. It hadn't come to me before, not like that. Would the thought have come to me, without pushing myself to see him like this? Perhaps not. I have discovered that when I pushed at life, things opened in strange ways. I did not know that before all this. *Application!*

I said goodbye.

On the way out, I spoke with the woman. I said thank you for taking care of him, and added that it seemed to me that someone had spent caring time. She seemed taken aback by this—my calmness? My recognition of the world around me at a time when it's perhaps more natural to be not cognizant of such? Even as I spoke I was so aware of the difference between a grieving person who has lost a beloved suddenly, shockingly, and someone like myself, who has already been grieving for months, who has had more sleep in the past three days than in the past three months, who is no longer in a state of panic.

Her guard was down; that happens when someone's work and effort is noticed. And she confided in me. "It was Ben, son of _____." She looked at me questioningly, and I nodded. I knew the man she was speaking of, leader of the local United church, a figure in the community. I laughed a bit, and then told her I knew this son, Ben, because he was a good friend of a young woman I knew, and they'd both been parts of a team of teens some years before who'd gathered at my home to dread my oldest son's hair when he was fourteen, and I'd plied them with pizza and sodas.

She stopped whispering. "Yes," she said. "We have meetings at which we decide which employee works with each individual. Ben asked to work with Marty."

I was so touched.

When I walked out, there was Ben, watering the flowers newly planted in the beds by the front door. Man of all trades, I suppose. Though watering flowers would be restorative work with what else he did. I thanked him directly. He was such a young man, I marvelled at the work he did. I was so glad I'd reached out with the compliment to the woman, and as a result learned who it was with such care.

122

Furniture and Friends

IN THE IMMEDIATE days after Marty died, the boys and I assembled the furniture. We needed it out of the house, with the sense that the sooner we could return to how our home used to be, the sooner we could remember Who Marty and Dad Was Before ALS. We needed that. Even the very afternoon, after the funeral home people had come and taken his body, after Cleve and Emmett went to fetch their grandparents, Ole and I moved the furniture into the entranceway.

I contacted the communications people a couple of days later, and they said we would be waiting for a while for them to come and collect the unusable iPad stand. I explained why we felt it would be good to have it out soon. It should have been either used or out weeks before. At which point, she made the suggestion that I disassemble, pack it up, and take it to nearest post office. "My husband died two days ago," I said. "You want me to... what?"

She repeated.

I hung up, shaking. A while later, I sent an email requesting them to please pick up the stand as quickly as possible.

Or they might find it at the foot of the driveway.

The assistant came along the next day, apologized, gave me a hug, took the stand apart, and packed it up and away. It was the last piece of equipment to leave the house.

Before the rest of the furniture was picked up, though— the bed, the chair, the shower commode, the hospital table—I stood in the midst of it, in moments of silence and respect. "You've each done your job." I touched the velour of the chair, and the metal of the bed rail. I remembered the cooling of that rail on my forehead when my sinus-infection pain was doing me in in those last weeks. I feared touching the chunky plastic of the shower chair, but I did; how I'd wrestled with that damn thing, how often it had had me in tears. I could still see my husband's thinned body on it, his deflated muscles, the paper thin of his ass cheeks, his slackened face, smile gone into lines, lines pulled. But without that chair, all would have been harder. The chair had allowed him to lie back, to sink into it, and have those times of some pleasure-of-sorts. Moments of something that looked like peace.

As I said goodbye to these pieces, I attempted to imbue them or bless them or... there was no instruction for this, just a sense that I must do this before letting them go to the next person. These pieces needed to be free of frustration, disappointment, resentment, sadness, and blessed with peace. I realized how silent the house was. Boys out or upstairs. Radio off. Television off. The sun was outside— it was spring after all—and streaming through windows. As if nothing had happened. Even though everything was finally changed. There was a strange sense of settling. Now life would go back to change at its usual pace, which was, for the most part, much slower. The tortoise is always the happier of the tortoise and hare. But it was forever changed.

One of the men came to pick up the pieces; the ALS Society employed two men to move and put together the furniture in our part of the world. I'd gotten to know both of them, a bit, between tidbits of conversation over the months. He looked sad, though not in a way that he really let me see. But I could. Did he ever get used to this? I suspected not. He shared with me that he'd made a first delivery to the home of a young man in his mid-twenties earlier that day. I asked him if the Society had anyone for him and his colleague to talk with; it had to be hard to do what they did. "No," he said. We exchanged a hug. I knew I'd never see him again, and that he would go on doing this work, and have cheering and real things to say to people, and then pass from their lives, moving on to the next, with respect and kindness. I hoped he had a good family, and a spouse at home, who gave him a hug when he walked in the door, and listened to his stories of his days, and perhaps the stories of her days could cause him to laugh now and again. I hoped he had a good friend.

123

Resurrecting Mary and Martha

IN THE DOWNSTAIRS living space, that one great room, there was a string of LED lights, red, gold, and green, that ran a couple of dozen feet, the length of the pine valance. They did not offer brightness, but just enough light not to have to turn on anything glaring through the night.

It was hospital headquarters with that enormous chair and the bed. Every time I sank into the bed's thick and supporting mattress, I was thankful. I was drifting in giant arms, holding me. It wasn't something I articulated at the time; it was just a sense. But I needed to pay attention to the sense, and to the rush of gratitude. Such moments—seconds really—changed the grinding reality. The seconds, through the days, created habit. So that allowing gratitude to sneak in, for simple things—which in fact seemed not so simple, hence the gratitude—was what made so much bearable.

After the time of readying Marty for bed, administering Ativan, attempting to sleep myself, at some point most nights there'd be a time of restlessness on his part. Insomnia would kick in, would overthrow the Ativan and wrestle sleep away from him. I'd be left with the sense that there was nothing I could do. There were no wrinkles in his clothing, for discomfort or pain, he was not hungry or thirsty. There was nothing on television. There needed to be some sleep, but sleep would not come. What to do?

His body was in pain. Muscles were deadened and heavy. Fasciculations had slowed, neurons had died. When I felt a slowed fasciculation, that thought came to me. It made it hard to touch him; I didn't like to feel fasciculations, and didn't like not to feel them. So it came to be that often in those last weeks, in the middle of the night, all that was left to me to do was to raise the footstool part of the recliner chair, and pull up one of the old kiddie chairs from the boys' set of table and chairs, wrap an afghan around my shoulders (Marty was so hot—unlike in the fall—with his body's natural thermostat no longer doing what it should, and we kept the house chilled). I would take off his socks, put some cream in my hands, something with a good smell to it, coconut or mango, something that smelled as if we should be in the sun somewhere, and then gently—very gently—rub his feet. It didn't take much for it to be too much. So I'd start with a general hand-warming, foot-warming rub, and then focus on the edges of his feet, working slowly, softly through each toe, the heels, the balls of his feet. My thoughts would drift. Over the past months. Then over the past years. I'd think about all the time we'd spent as a couple of people who lived under the same roof, but had little to say to each other. About happier times, times of feeling close. I'd think of sexually charged times, and then the foot rub would become more sensual, less about just making him feel sleepy and more about both of us feeling good.

There were two or three times when my mind drifted—
the exhausted mind of the caregiver—to words of the old
South Asian man who taught yoga at our local leisure centre.
His words: "We die from the feet up." He would say this
every Monday night as he had everyone in the class massage our own feet. He would urge us not to neglect our feet,
but to spend daily time caring for them, massaging them,
separating toes, running thumbs along the bottom, through
the centre.

At that point, it had been many months since I'd been to
one of those Monday classes, but the old man's words stayed
with me, and came to me then, in the middle of the night.

Too, that less-told story returned to me, from the book of
John: Martha going out into the town to find Jesus after her
brother Lazarus has died. She was so purposeful. Tenacious.
Martha's belief made her feet move. Something in her made
her dream and not accept. I'd never seen her actions in this
way before. And what did it mean, that Mary chose not to
go out, but to stay home and grieve?

Rubbing feet. Moving feet. My mind roved in the middle
of the night.

I massaged my thumbs into Marty's insteps, and my
mind looped back to the early days of diagnosis, back to that
window of time of hope, looking for answers, the belief that
seemed to have arisen from some deep thought that there
had to be some escape from this, if only we, or I, could find
it, find the key. All the crazy shit out there in the world,
about toxins and natural healing and possibilities. In those
middle-of-the-night—deep into the night—times, I would
find myself, uncensored (too tired to think), wondering
about the possibility that this could be It: that if one was to

spend hours—the bulk of the day really—massaging, pulling the body's toxins down down down into one's feet, and then drawing them out, that somehow this could be it. Imagine! ALS solved. It was just a matter of hours. And doing. And hours. And more doing. Dedication. Love. Feeling it through and through and pulling out all the Bad Stuff so that healing could take place. I'd find suddenly that it had indeed been about an hour that I was there, sitting on a child-sized chair, kneading. My heart, which had felt heavy through the day, lightened with a feeling of well-being—brought about by what? Giving? And somehow the illogical would have a sense of making sense. How did that work? Just with the slowing? Sense of care? His stillness? My own lack of sleep bringing on a certain madness? Somehow the irritating drone of the ever-present podcast would recede, and I'd feel as if it just didn't matter. Nothing mattered, except the connecting of feet and hands, and the moment. If it didn't heal him, it was healing me. For the moment. The moment was enough.

What we are left with under the stars. For now.

124.

Summer 2017

MONTHS HAVE PASSED. More than a year. Many moments.

I have just sold my home. I've bought one half of a duplex, which is about half of the square footage of the home we have lived in, but in the city, close to music, to festivals, to places to savour food and drink and human beings. I've gone to the city's jazz festival, to fireworks, to restaurants new to me, to small music venues. I've continued to dance, and almost weekly find music to dance to. Blues, R&B, funk. Klezmer even. Really? An accordion-noir festival? Who knew?

I dance often, when I go to hear music. I've begun to play my dad's old saxophone, the instrument that he—with his ALS now—can no longer play. I had never been able to get a sound out of it, in spite of several tries when I was much younger. Not until now. It sounds not bad. I play "When Sunny Gets Blue." And "When I Fall In Love." So many whens. Maybe more ifs.

I walk into my backyard, thinking how I have signed the papers that mean this space is in fact someone else's backyard now.

I look at the deck, the chiminea, retired to a corner and

filled with candles as tribute to fire and warmth. I've gotten rid of so much furniture indoors and out, including the large table and chairs on which we used to share food out here. There is no room for them at the new place. There, there'll be room only for the wicker pieces, and the crescent-shaped footstool on which to warm toes in front of the propane fireplace. There will be that. When we eat, we'll eat on our laps. It will be good.

I feel the grass under my bare feet, and realize that this may be the last time in my life I own grass. I wonder if it's even right that we can own grass. In my new home there is a tiny stone courtyard with ocean waves of traffic outside the fence, and there is a corner shade garden full of green to which I need to add colour. I will hang my wind-chimes— the musical thin pipes, and the chunking bamboo. I see myself there, with a glass of wine, and a friend, or with my boys, talking, listening to music. Laughing. Sharing. Being people together. That's what we have. Right now.

Behind me, boxes are full, taped, labelled. Ready.

For this moment, I feel the grass, prickling and poking between my toes, as if someone is rubbing my feet, breathing sun-warmth and life into them. I am so glad to be here, in this place.

Someday, all heaven's going to break loose. Martha's going to rise up and dance as never before, and as no one has seen. She's going to lift her sister Mary from where she's kneeling, and together they'll dance, conjoined, in recognition of a moment of simple happiness.

Acknowledgements

FROM THE TIME written of in these pages, I thank our family doctor, Dr. David Kason, who was with us from that first day. And in the journey that followed—the writing of these pages—there was the wisdom of Andreas Schroeder, one of a small number of early readers who read with care, each with a different and useful perspective; for this I am grateful.

And then there are the many individuals—dozens or more—who were with us through those months: family members who renovated and cooked and cleaned, who came with foot bath and electric blanket, flowers, and love; friends and neighbours who brought laughter and food— everything from lasagne to popovers, to fruit and tea; those who brought books and paint chips, and those who sent cards and messages; those who took care of the garden, pruned and raked.

Some picked up and drove friends from the airport, and some traveled to visit; still others came on a break in their day, with lunch. There were the other medical practitioners—all did their best. There was a carer who assisted with showers through the week, one who offered therapeutic touch, and another with silver fabric to wind between raw fingers . . . such detail.

To those who organized the Party for Marty, and raised funds, played music, took care of the food, the silent auction, the cleaning, and to those who spent evenings with Marty, watching hockey and golf while I danced, and to all the aforementioned people and more: I thank each and all of you from the deepest place in my heart.

Thank you to the team at Brindle & Glass, and to my agent, for your belief and passion.

Have I forgotten someone? Some deed? Many acts and gifts were done and given—so many that I am not convinced I can ever fully know. So much was quietly taken care of by the nameless and loving who sought no accolades or acknowledgement. I thank them as well.

ALISON ACHESON is the author of ten books, including the short story collection *Learning to Live Indoors* (Porcupine's Quill), which was praised by the *Globe & Mail* for its "arresting and crystalline clarity". She teaches creative writing at the University of British Columbia, and lives in Vancouver, BC.

Permissions